Universal Chi Kids
Smiling Anatomy for Children

Level I
for ages 5 -7

Mantak Chia
&
Sarina Stone

Edited by:

Suthisa Chaisarn

Editor: Suthisa Chaisarn

Illustrations: Udon Jandee

Computer Graphics: Hiranyathorn Pansan

Production Manager: Suthisa Chaisarn

First published in 2010
ISBN: 978-0-9826384-0-8

Contents

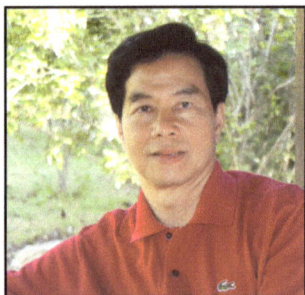

Grand Master Mantak Chia

Grand Master Mantak Chia is the creator of the Universal Healing Tao System and the director of the Tao Garden Health Resort in the beautiful northern countryside of Thailand. Since childhood he has been studying the Taoist approach to life. His mastery of this ancient knowledge, enhanced by his study of natural health, has resulted in the development of the Universal Healing Tao System which is now being taught throughout the world.

Mantak Chia was born in Thailand to Chinese parents in 1944. When he was six years old, Buddhist monks taught him how to sit and "still the mind." While still a grammar school student, he learned traditional Thai boxing. He was then taught Tai Chi Chuan by Master Lu, who soon introduced him to Aikido, Yoga and broader levels of Tai Chi.

Grand Master Chia is a great lover of family values and children and is very proud to bring this special Smiling Anatomy to children around the world.

Sarina Stone

Sarina Stone is a Certified Universal Healing Tao Instructor and Director of Chi Kids Incorporated, a non-profit corporation dedicated to educating families and children about natural health through art and literature.

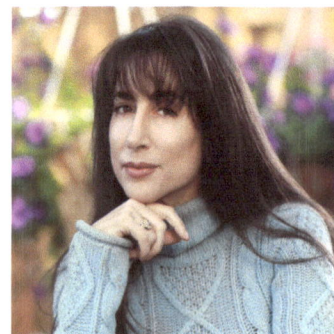

Her study of Eastern Chi Kung, Western natural health, and stress relief methods has provided the basis for her lighthearted approach to the often complicated field of wellness and self-realization. These user-friendly methods have made her an internationally sought after speaker, author and Medical Chi Kung instructor. Her lectures have been made available through the internet, various schools and Universities as well as several guest spots on both radio and television. It is her sincere hope that the material contained in these children's books aid youth in making healthy choices and creating abundant health.

For more information, go to www.sarinastone.com

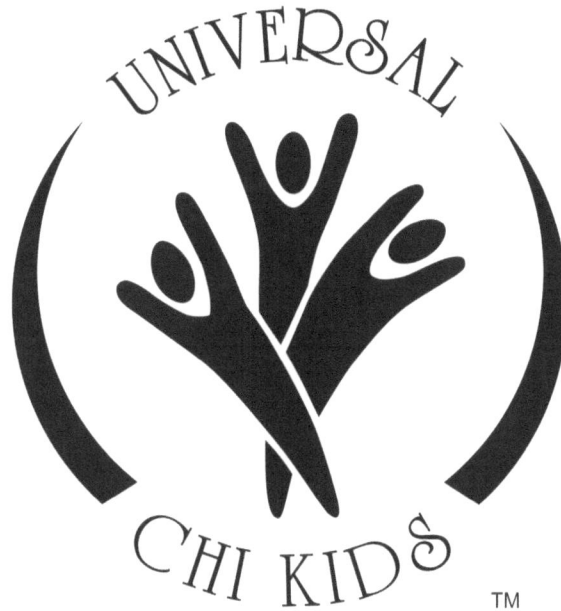

Chi Kids and Universal Chi Kids

Helping Kids To Help Themselves

Chi Kids Incorporated is a non-profit, 501.c.3 corporation dedicated to teaching children and families about natural health through art and literature. Universal Chi Kids is a trademark of Chi Kids Incorporated.

Chi Kids Incorporated, in partnership with Grand Master Mantak Chia and Universal Healing Tao, is proud to announce the first line of products designed to teach young kids and their grown-ups these unique stress relief and self awareness techniques. Chi Kids families are proactive families; therefore these products are designed to be experienced by grown-ups and children together. Please take this opportunity and spend some "quality" time with a young person and utilize this amazing system to learn about yourself and each other.

A NOTE FROM SARINA STONE

*As an adolescent, do you think some of your emotional choices would have been different if you **truly believed** that spending long periods of time in states of worry and anxiety would cause illnesses like colds, flu and even acne?*

*As a young adult, is there even a chance you may have walked away earlier from intensely negative or toxic situations if you **truly believed** that they might cause tumors and even premature death?*

If this were what you truly believed today, wouldn't you share that knowledge with your child to help prevent illness into their adult life?

Once upon a time, thousands of years ago, mystical sages taught secret practices for health and longevity to the emperors of China. It is known that these emperors were super human in their wisdom and strength. They were heralded as the greatest leaders of their time. Today, through the teachings of people like Taoist Master, Mantak Chia, these secrets are available for you and your family.

Some of these techniques, or "formulas" are deceivingly simple.
For example, the power of a Smile is greatly under-rated in many parts of the world. And yet, western doctors acknowledge that sadness and depression inhibit the immune system and in some severe cases may even cause death. If the ailment were sadness and depression, would the preventative medicine not be joyfulness? I assure you, a Smile is far less expensive than a prescription drug and no one has ever damaged their organs, gone through withdrawal or gotten the strength of their Smile dangerously wrong.

Smiling Chi (energy) Kung (work) has its roots in ancient *Taoist medicine and has been used in China for more than 5000 years. Taoist meditation may be used as a means to understand the true human potential and connect with, feel and ultimately control the systems of the body. Once mastered, the practitioner may then utilize the awesome power of the mind to attain physical health and emotional balance, EVEN IF THEY ARE 5 YEARS OLD!

It has been my experience that young, open-minded people are far more adept at mastering these techniques than those who have developed notions of right and wrong, possible and impossible. Children know that any thing they imagine becomes real. So let us be responsible grown-ups and teach them that good health and a peaceful mind are just Smiles away.

* Chinese to English translation of the word Tao – The Way of Nature, The Way Without Force, The Way

Yours in Tao,
Sarina Stone

Acknowledgements

Sarina and Master Chia wish to thank the following for their kind contributions:

All the wonderful children and families who posed for photos.
Thank you for patiently waiting while we edited these books!

R. Mordant Mahon for line editing while he was attending instructor training.

Anthony Andaloro for artistic direction and photography.

Udon Jandee for amazing cartoons.

Hirunyathorn Punsan for production support.

Universal Healing Tao for their kindness, wisdom and unlimited support.

Chi Kids Incorporated for undying faith in the wisdom of children.

A very special thank you to all those parents who let their kids color outside of the lines.

Chapter 1
Heart Sound

Recommended for ages 5-7
I can Smile to my Heart

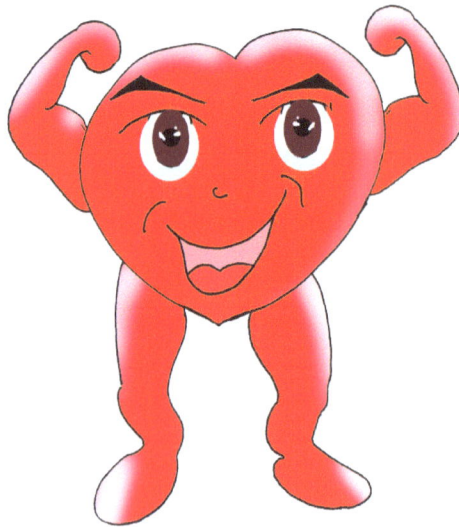

Inner Smile & Sounds That Heal

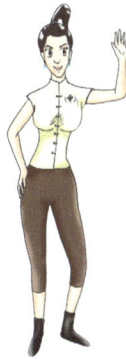

Welcome to Chi Kids "I Can Smile To My Heart" Level I.
My name is Sarina.
I am very excited to share this magic formula with you.
My teacher, Master Smile, taught me how to smile to my Heart a long time ago
and now I am going to share with you.

Once you learn this secret, be sure to teach it to someone else!
We call this special magic Chi Kung.

Chi is energy and Kung is work, so Chi Kung means "energy work" in Chinese.
Do you know anyone who speaks Chinese?

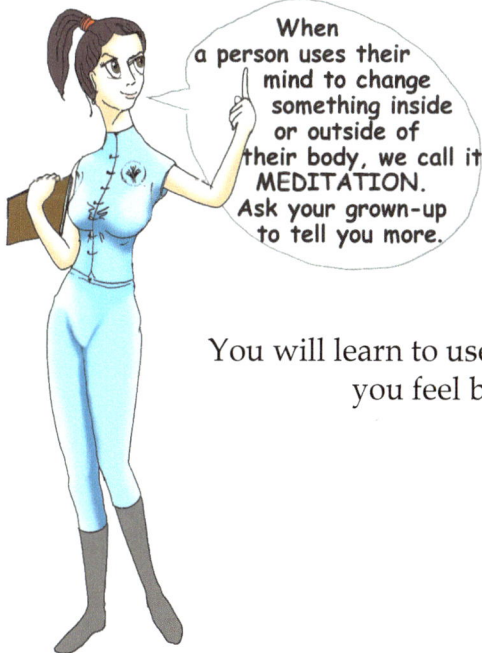

When a person uses their mind to change something inside or outside of their body, we call it MEDITATION. Ask your grown-up to tell you more.

This chapter will teach you where your Heart is, how to Smile to it, how to talk to it and how to make yourself feel happier just by thinking happy thoughts.

You will learn to use your own energy to help you feel better when you feel bad and be a happy, healthy person.

I'M A CHI KID

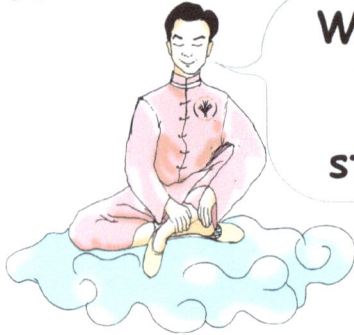

We are going to take a magical adventure inside our body. All you need to get started is a great big smile.

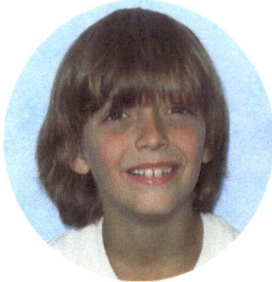

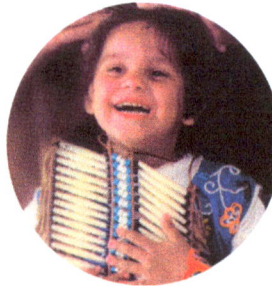

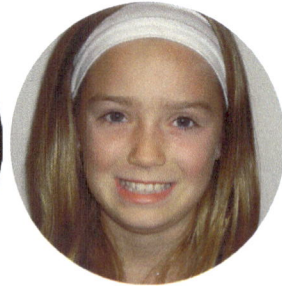

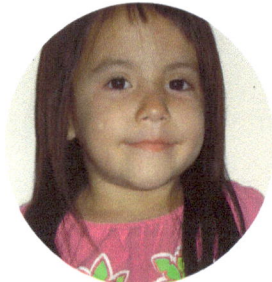

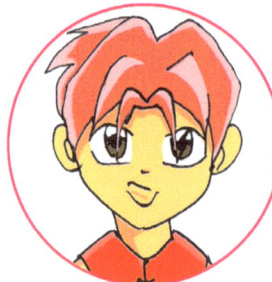

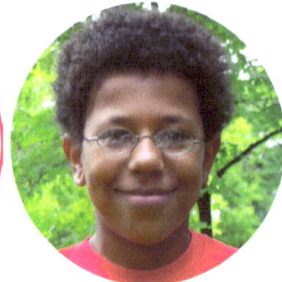

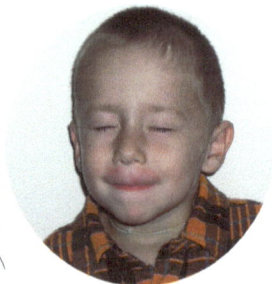

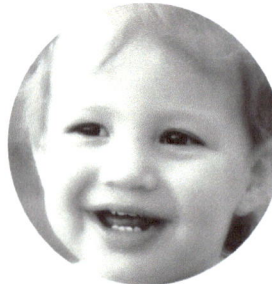

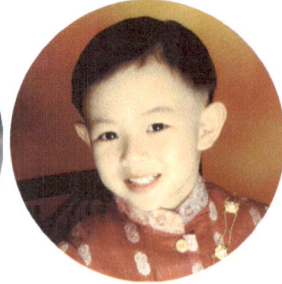

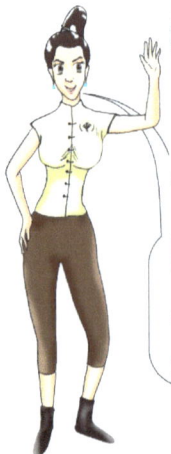

Look everyone. Its Master Smile! Smile real big and you will see him smile back!

3

You have a body.
You are the only person in the whole world born
with your body.

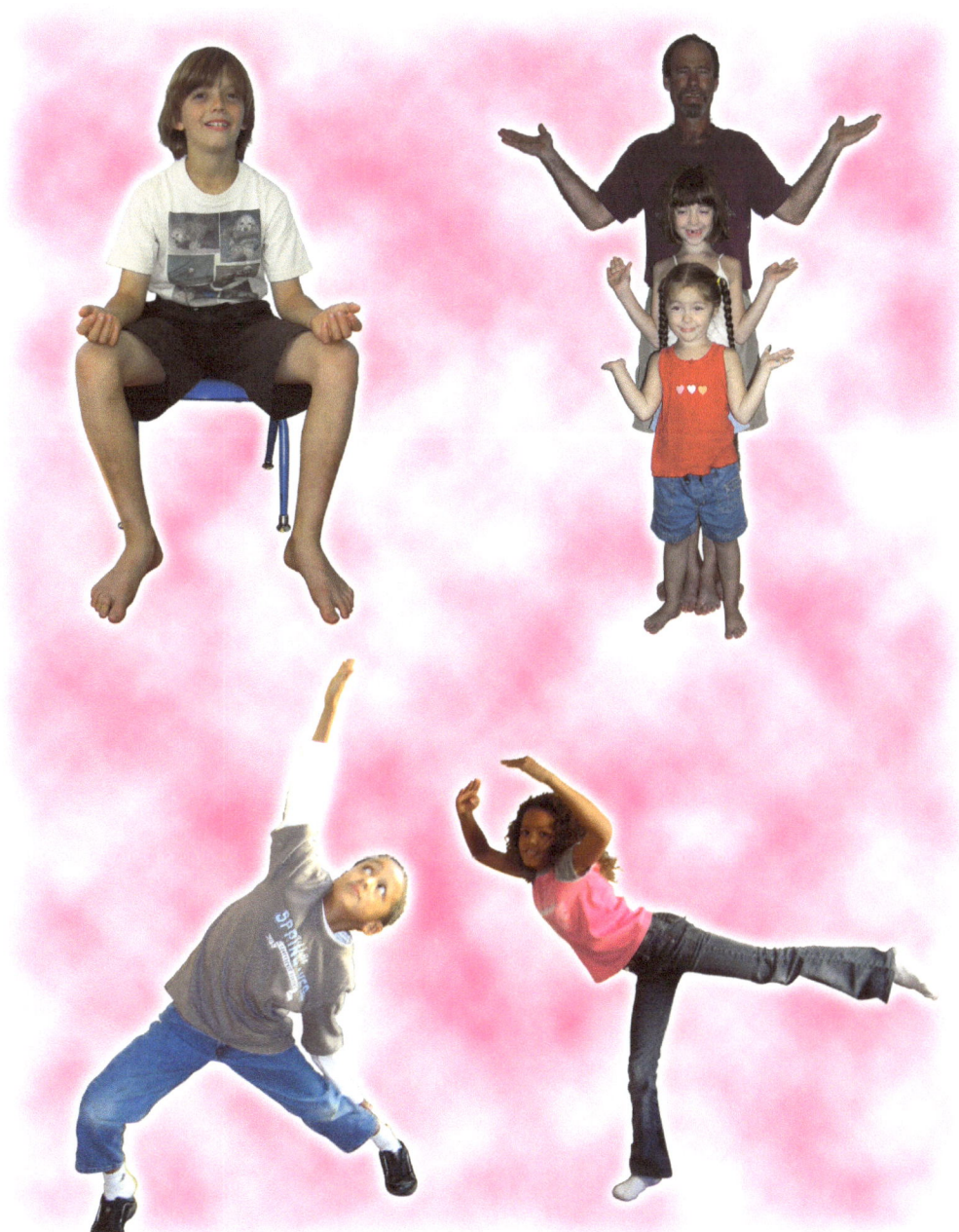

That makes you very special.

Your body has many parts.
Some parts are outside.

Outside

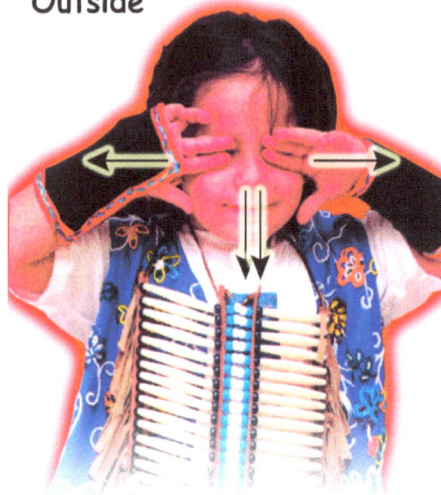

Some parts are inside.

Inside

Red   for the Heart
White   for the Lungs
Gold   for the Spleen
Blue   for the Kidneys
Green   for the Liver

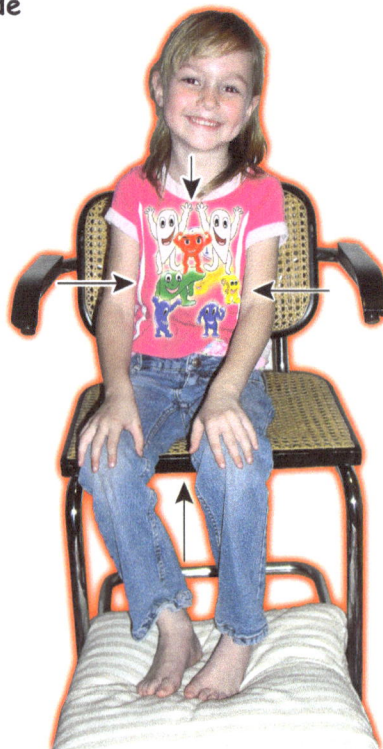

Today we will learn how to talk to your Heart.
And your Heart will learn to talk to you!!!!

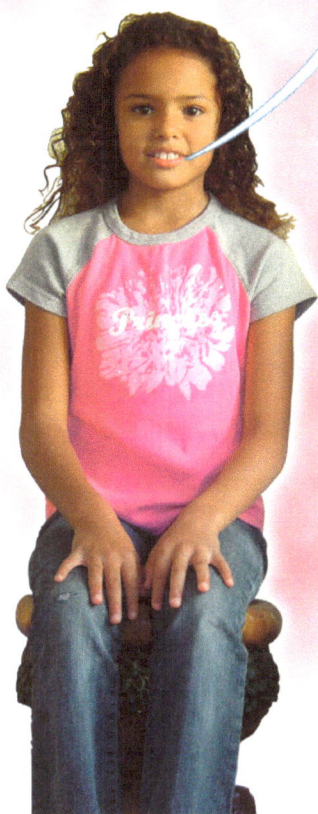
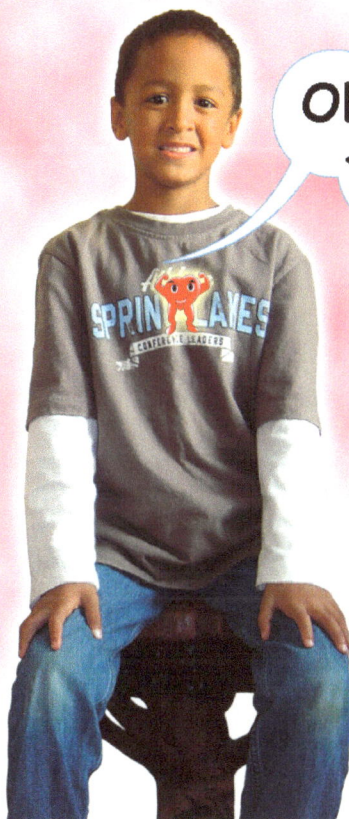

We begin by sitting in a chair with our feet on the ground
and feeling where our Heart is.
If you are very quiet, you will feel where your Heart is.

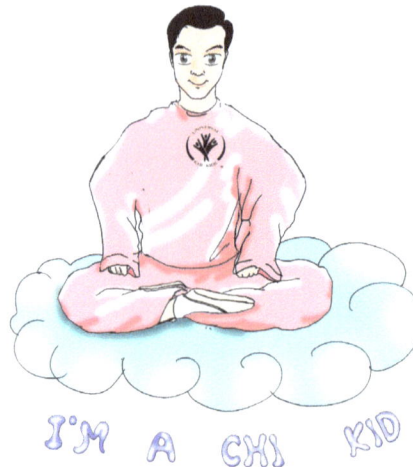

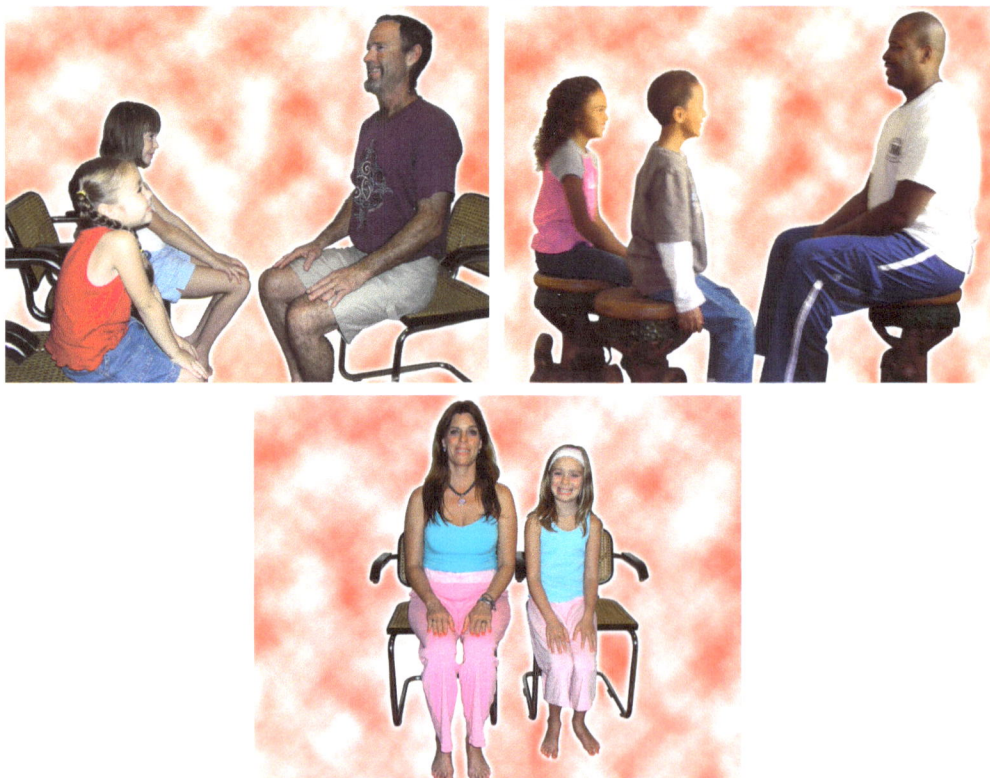

I'M A CHI KID

Ask your grown up for help finding the "thump-thump" feeling on the
left side of your chest. Then, ask your grown up what the Heart does for
you and your blood.

Now, here is the most important step.
Put a BIG smile on your face!

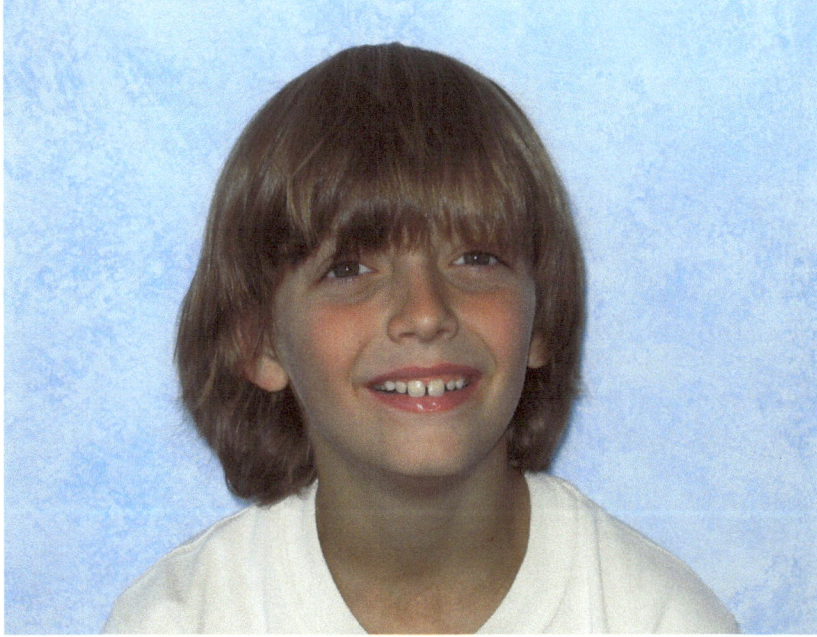

Smile to your Heart. Let your Heart smile back!

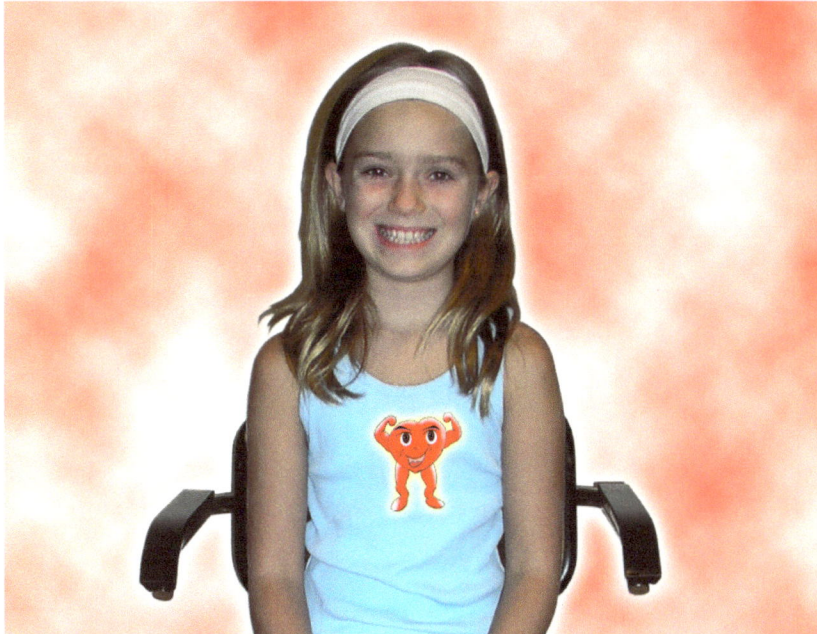

Close your eyes, smile to your Heart and breathe in the feeling of Love until you fill your beautiful Red Heart with the red color of Love.

Breathe out the feeling of Hate & Cruelty. See a dark smoke leave through your mouth and drop down into the earth.

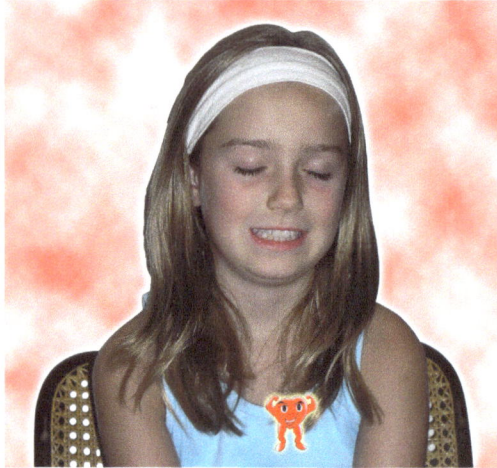

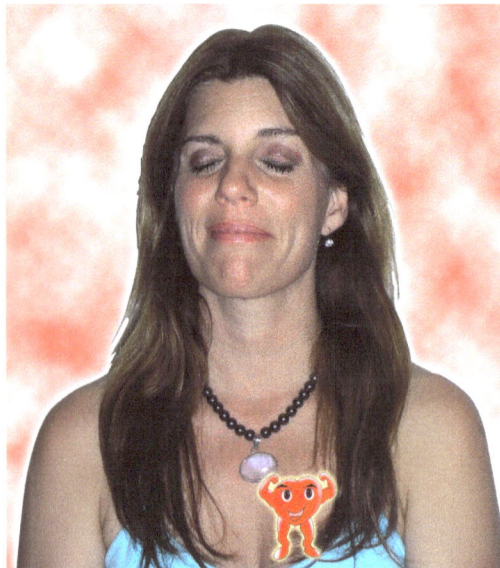

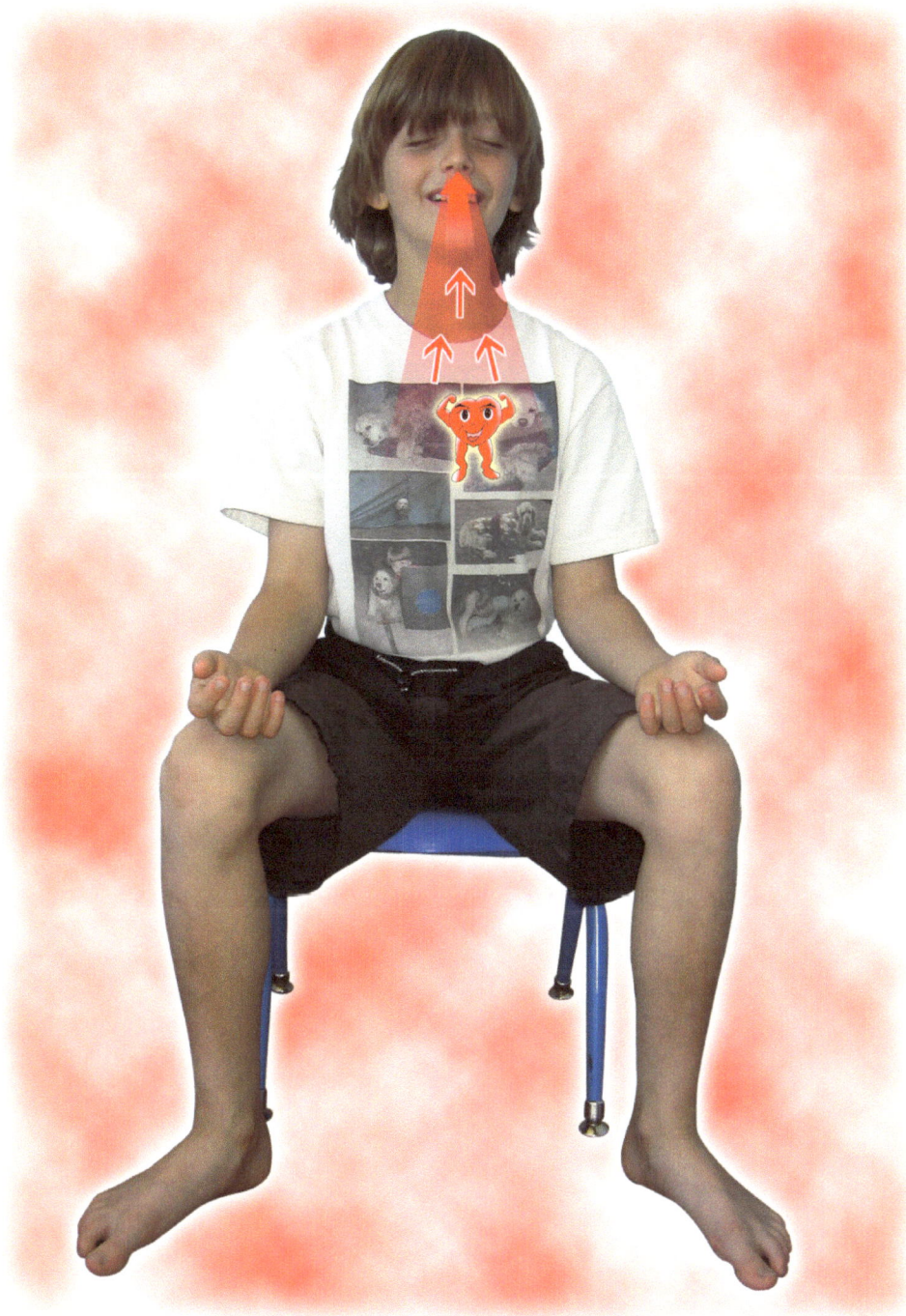

The Earth will take your garbage and use it to grow beautiful things, like flowers or trees. We call that TRANSFORMATION

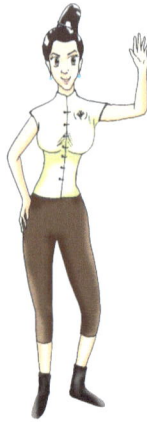

"Wow! That's a big word."

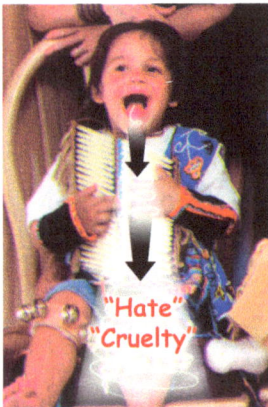

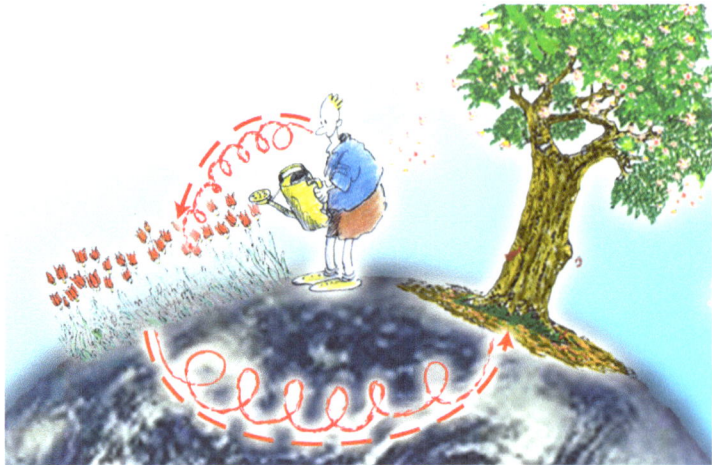

Smile to your big, Red, Loving Heart.

Lets try it again. This time, we're going to speak to our Heart out loud!
The special healing sound of the Heart is HAWWW

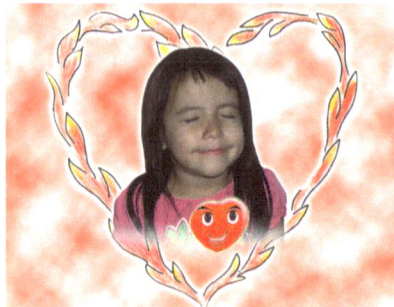

11

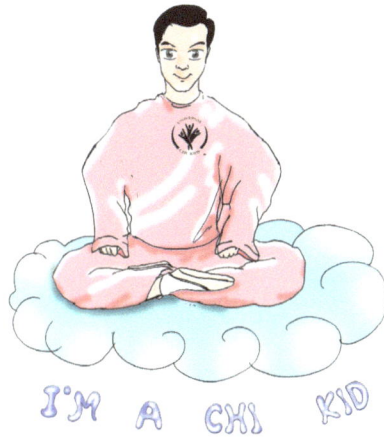

I'M A CHI KID

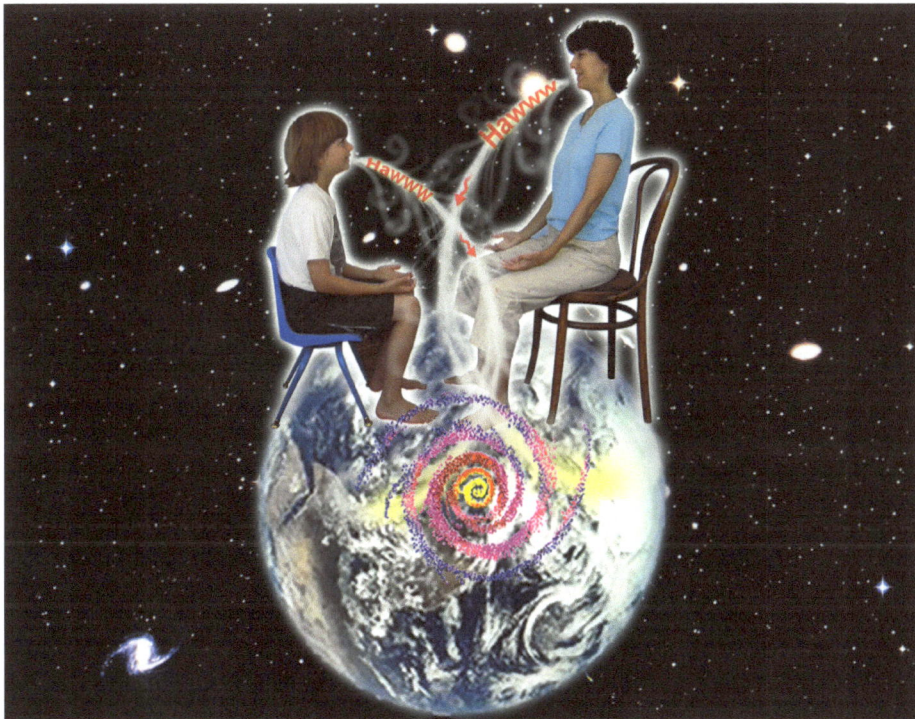

Can you say Hawww?

So, now we're going to breathe in love and breathe out Hate & Cruelty using the HAWWW sound. Remember to breathe out the dark smoke and let it go into the Earth.

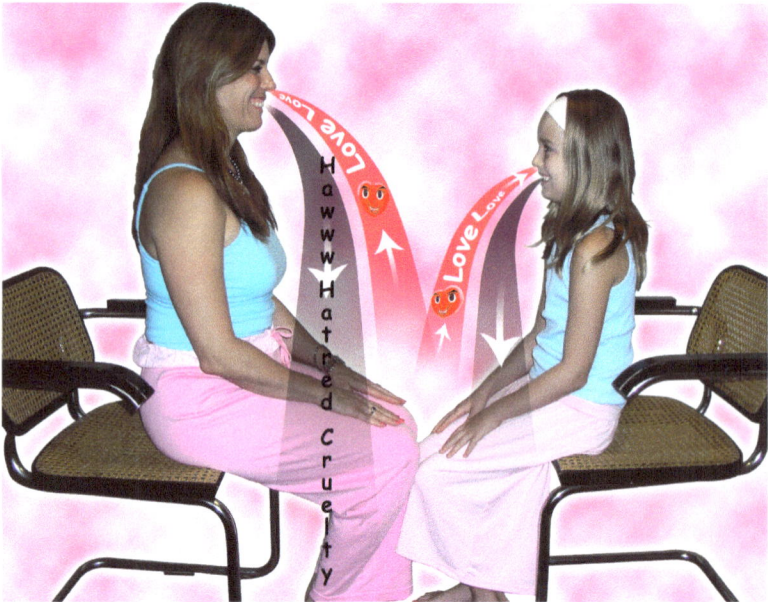

Are you still smiling?
You should be!

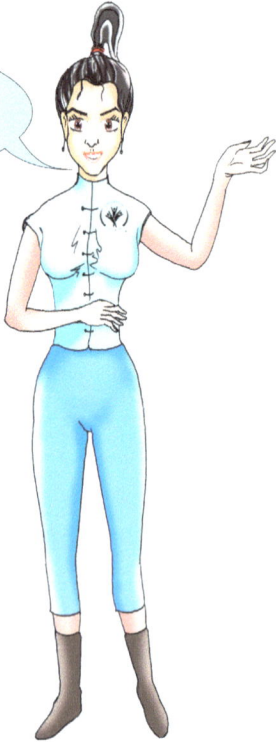

Look who's here! It's the Red Pheasant!
The Red Pheasant is like a guardian angel for your Heart.

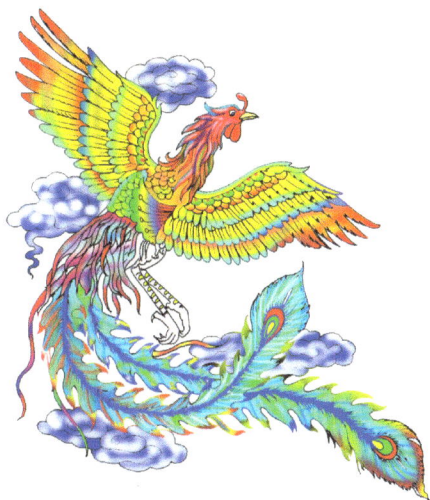

In the Taoist way, we believe there are special animals
to protect us from harm. When you smile to your Red Heart,
smile to the Red Pheasant too!

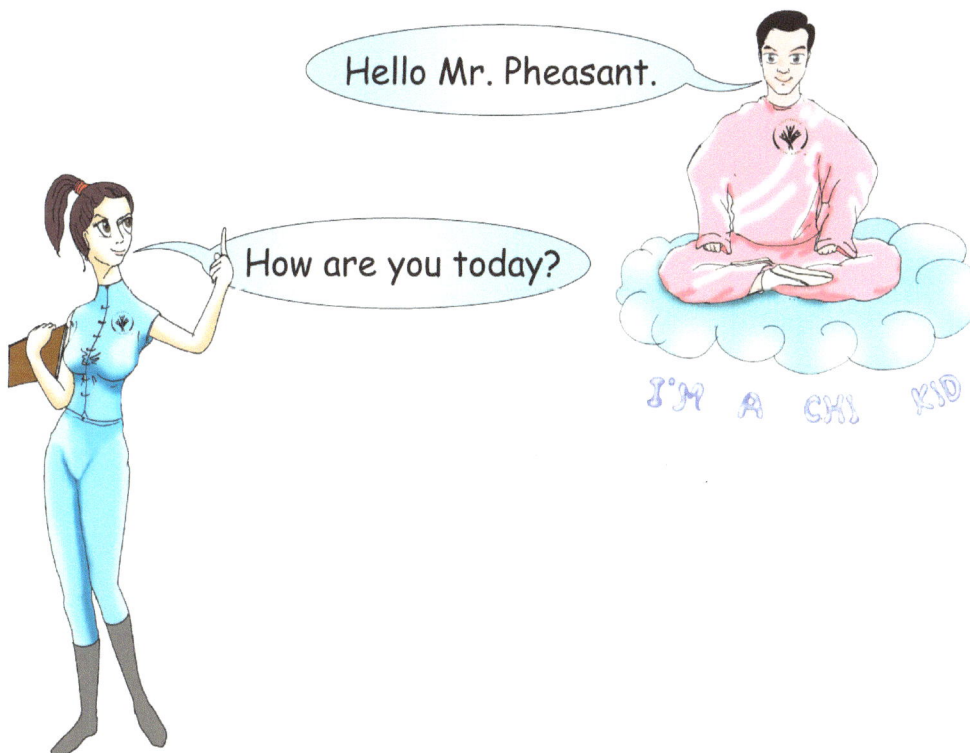

Hello Mr. Pheasant.

How are you today?

I'M A CHI KID

Let's put it all together!
Sit on a chair with your feet on the floor and SMILE.
Feel your Heart and Smile to your Heart.
See your Red Heart smile back.
Think about something or someone you love and breathe in
Love to your Heart.
Breathe out hatred & cruelty using the HAWW sound.
Let dark smoke leave your Heart through your mouth and imagine it
sinks into the earth. The Earth can use it to grow something beautiful.
Say "Hello" to the Red Pheasant that protects your Heart.
Smile one more time and feel the Loving feeling coming
from your Heart.

Try to do this 3 times in a row!

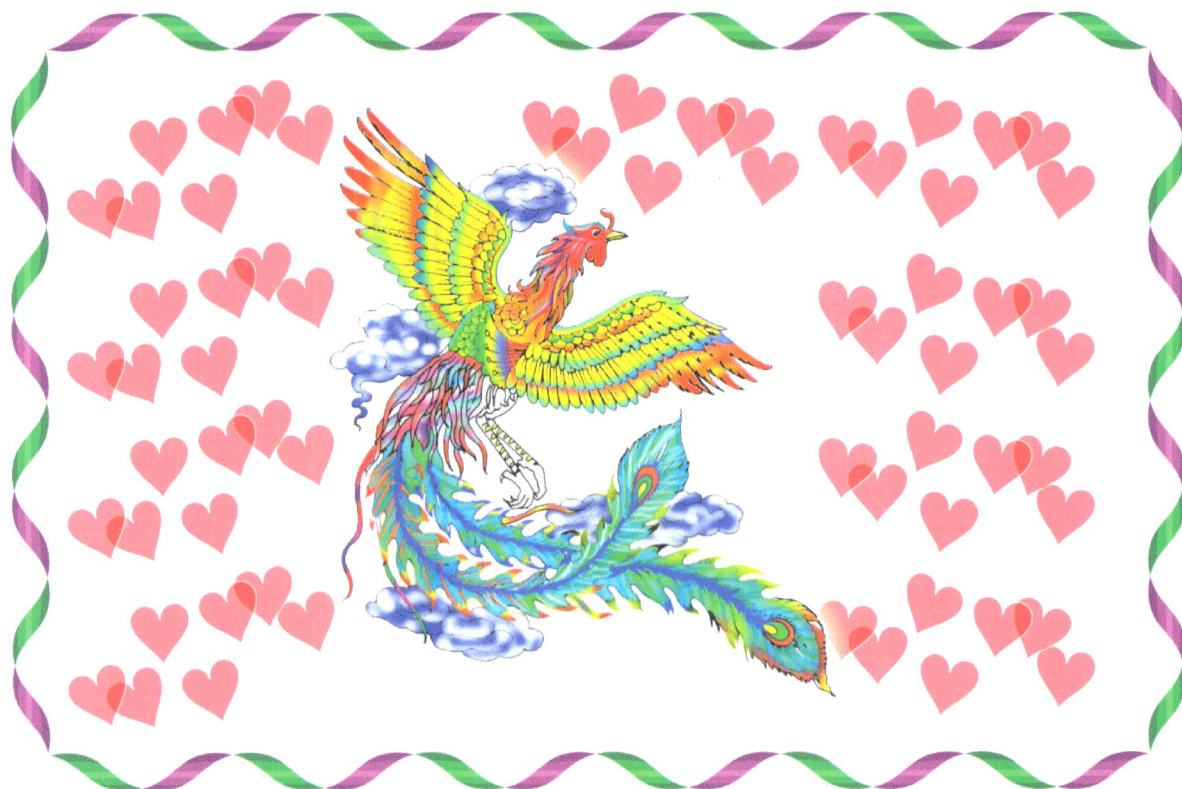

It is always important to take a minute and
rest after we Smile to our Heart.
Just take one or two minutes and think of all the people you love,
and the people who love you.

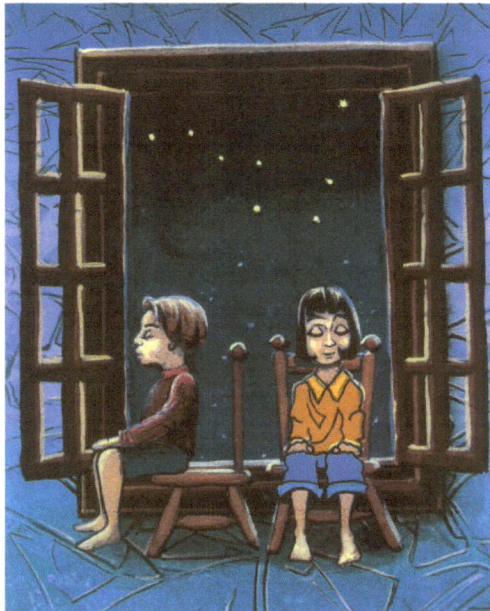

And, remember, to love yourself.

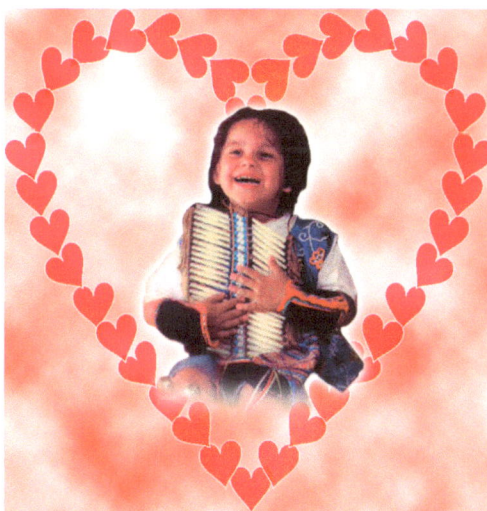

You are a very special person!

Chapter 2
Lungs Sound

Recommended for ages 5-7
I can Smile to my Lungs

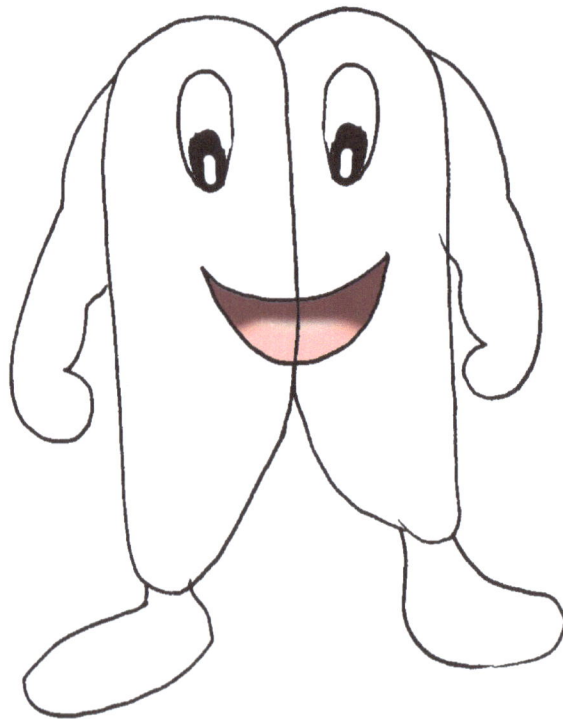

Inner Smile & Sounds That Heal

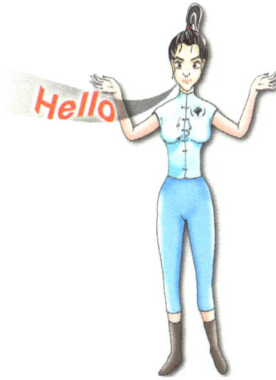

Welcome to Chi Kids "I Can Smile To My Lungs" Level I. My name is Sarina.
I am very excited to share this magic formula with you. My teacher, Master Smile,
taught me how to smile to my Lungs a long time ago and now I am going to share with
you. Once you learn this secret, be sure to teach it to someone else!

Remember, we call this special magic Chi Kung. Chi is energy and Kung is work,
so Chi Kung means "energy work" in Chinese.

This chapter will teach you where your LUNGS are, how to SMILE to them, how to
TALK to them and how to make yourself feel happier just by thinking happy thoughts.

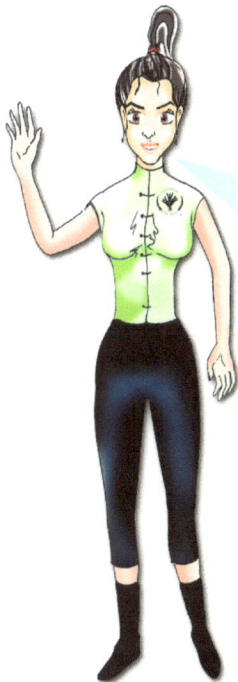

When a person uses their mind
to change something inside or
outside of their body, we call
it MEDITATION. Ask your
grown-up to tell you more.

You will learn to use your own energy to help
you feel better when you feel bad and be a happy,
healthy person.

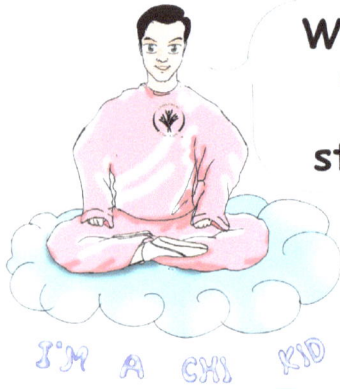

We are going to take a magical adventure inside our body. All you need to get started is a great big smile.

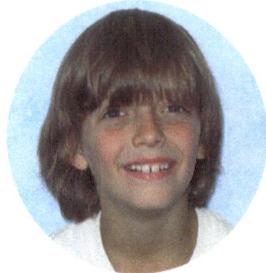

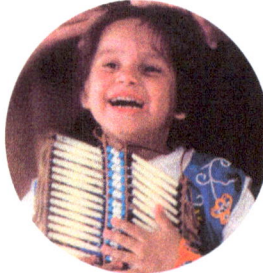

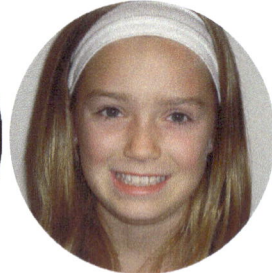

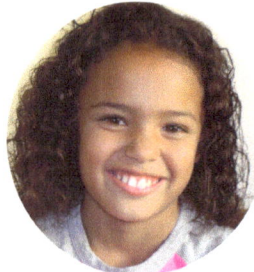

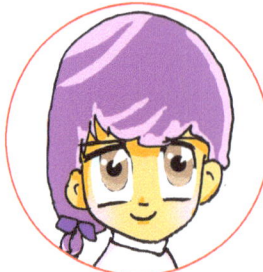

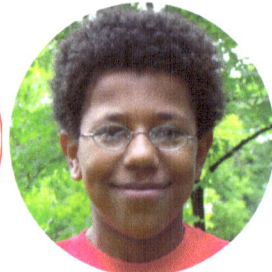

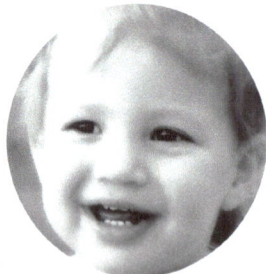

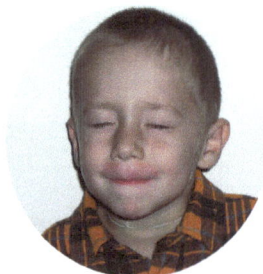

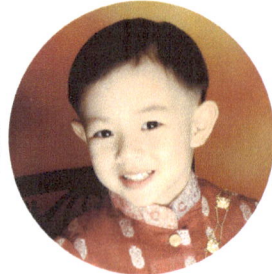

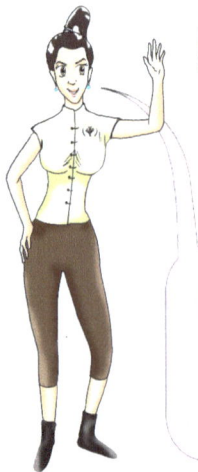

I'M A CHI KID

Look everyone! It's Master Smile! Smile real big and you will see him smile back!

21

You have a body.
You are the only person in the whole world born with your body.

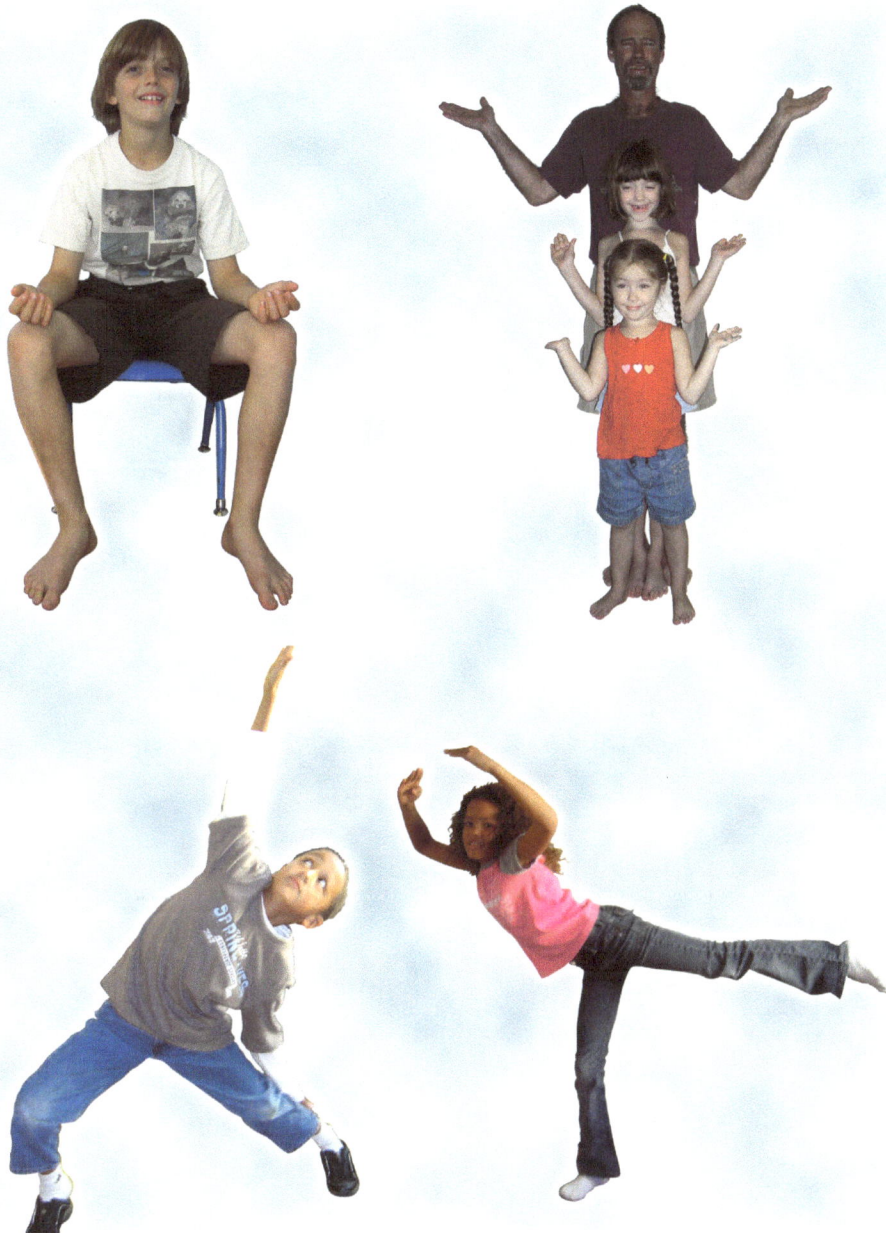

That makes you VERY special.

Your body has many parts.
Some parts are outside.
Some parts are inside.

Inside

Outside

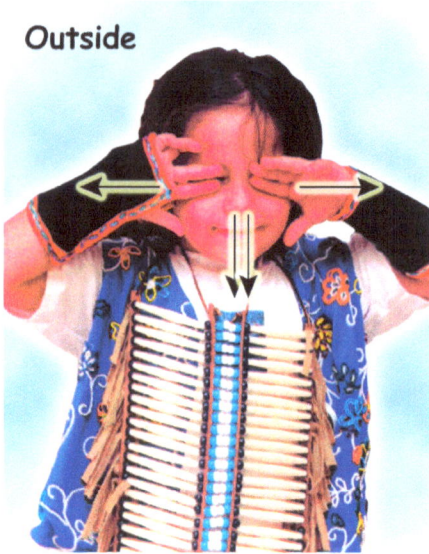

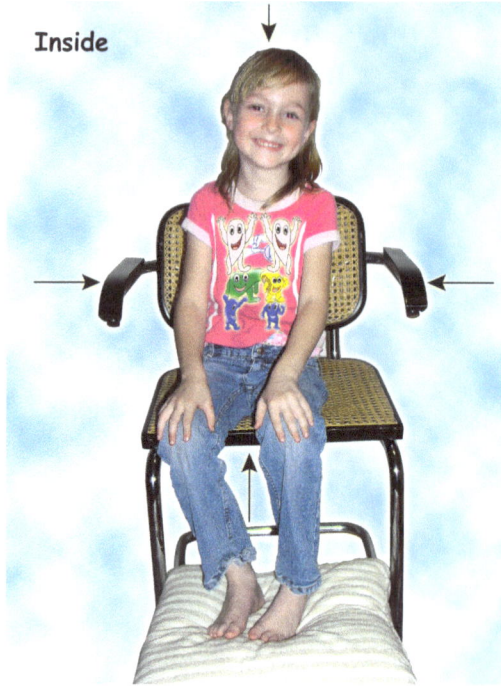

Today we will learn how to talk to your Lungs and your Lungs
will learn to talk to you!!!!

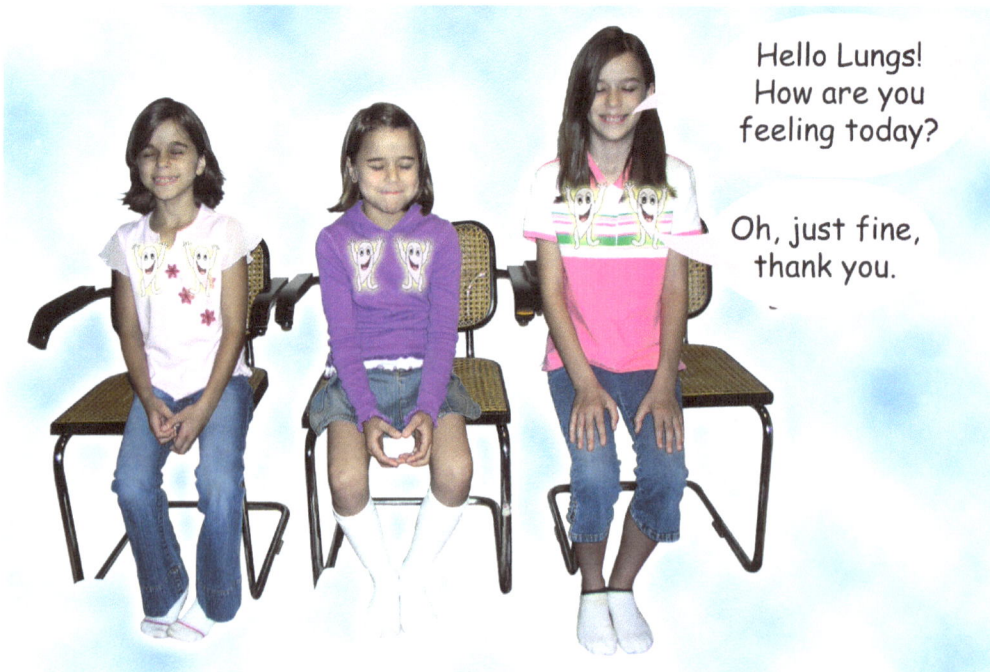

Hello Lungs!
How are you
feeling today?

Oh, just fine,
thank you.

Begin by sitting on a chair with your feet on the ground.
Then, be quiet and FEEL where your Lungs are.

Take a deep breath into your chest. Your chest gets bigger because your lungs are filling with air! Ask your grown up what the lungs do for you and how they help you breath.

I'M A CHI KID

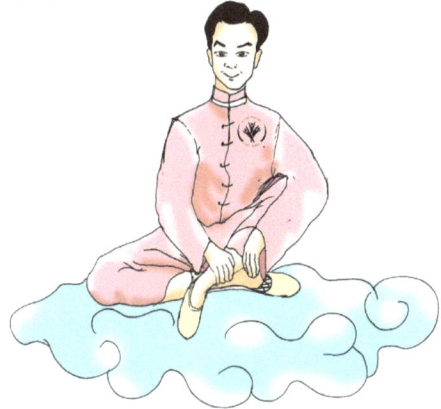

Here is a picture to help you find them.

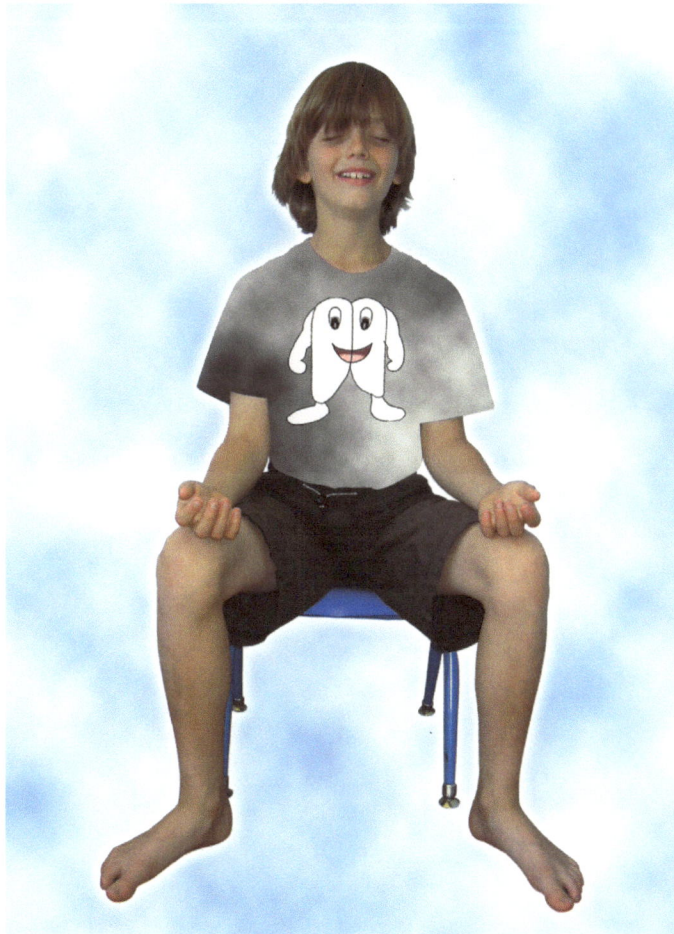

Put a BIG smile on your face!
Take a deep breath and Smile to your Lungs.

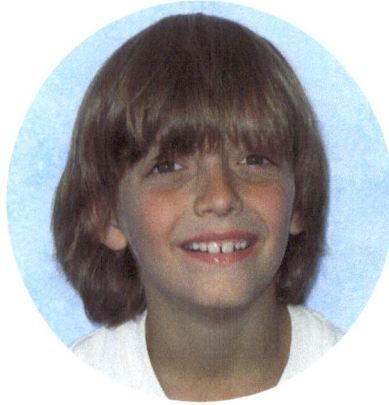

Let your Lungs smile back!
Be sure to breathe out when you're finished!!

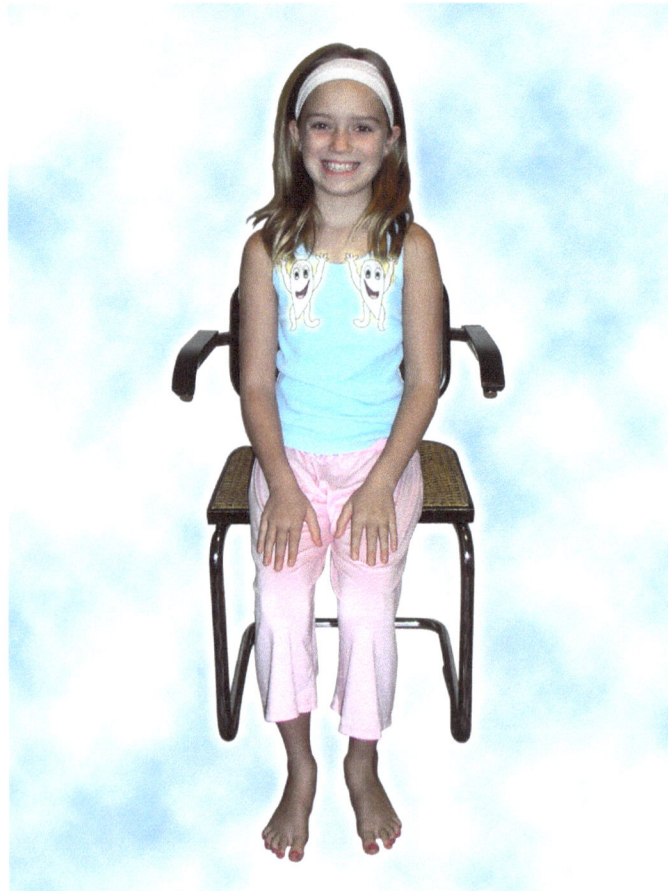

Imagine your Lungs as a beautiful White color.

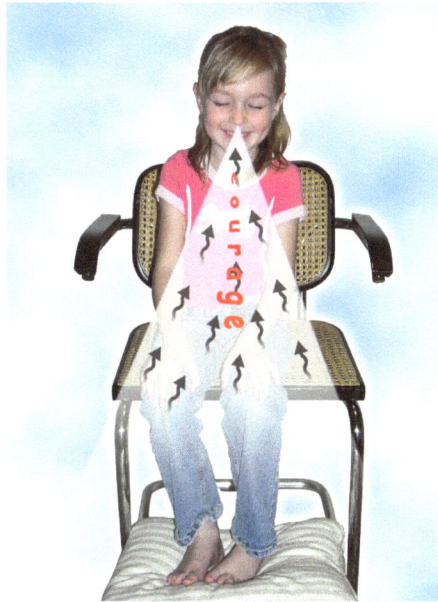

Close your eyes, Smile to your Lungs and
breathe in the feeling of Courage.
Fill your beautiful White Lungs with Courage.

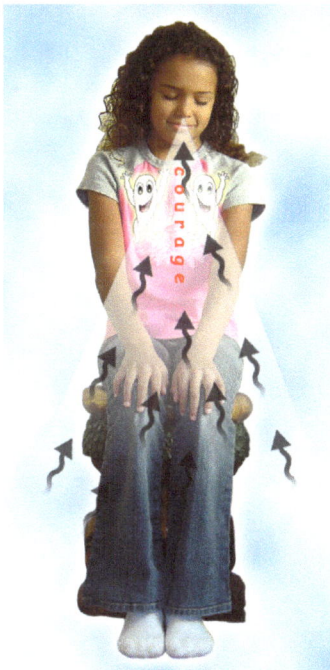

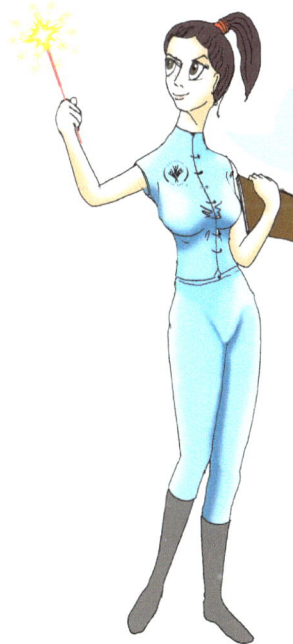

Good work!
Your lungs are
smiling already!

Breathe out the feeling of Sadness.
See a dark smoke leave through
your mouth and drop down into the
earth.

The Earth will take your sadness and
use it to grow beautiful things like
flowers and trees.

I'M A CHI KID

Bye-bye sadness
Hello flowers

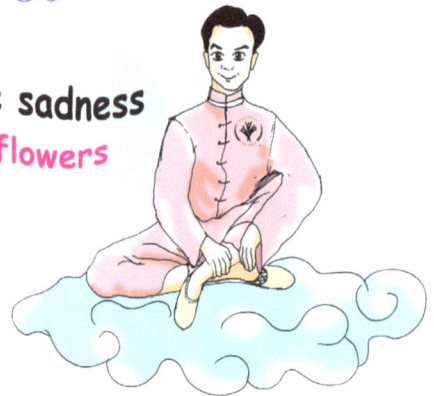

We call that TRANSFORMATION.

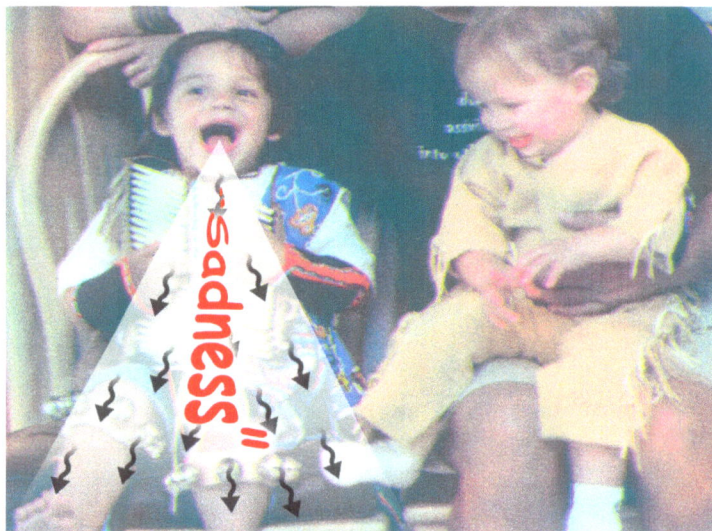

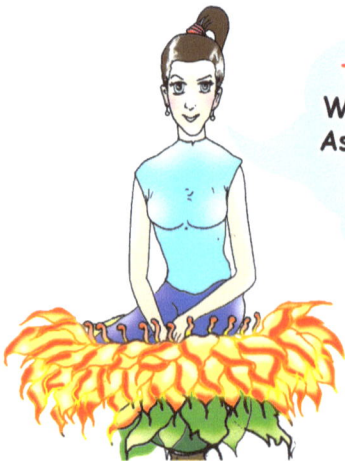

sadness

TRANSFORMATION.
Wow! That's a big word.
Ask your grown-up about
that big word.
Bye-bye **sadness**
Hello flowers.

Smile to your shiny White Courageous Lungs.

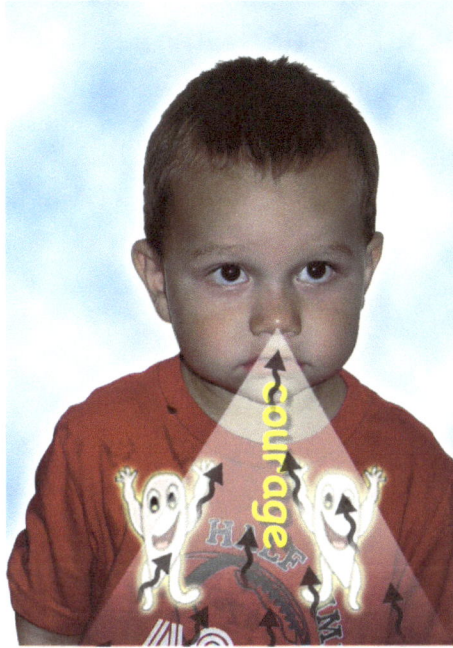

This little boy needs to practice smiling.
Let's smile to him and help!

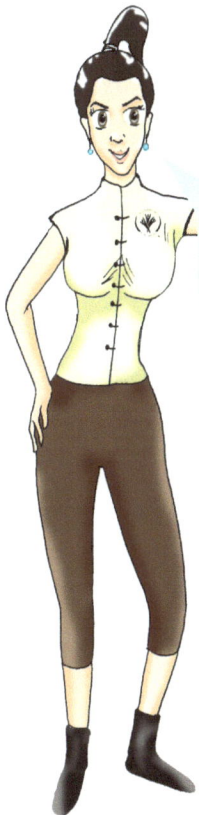

Can you say
SSSSSS?

Lets try it again. This time, we're going to
speak to our Lungs out loud!
The special HEALING sound of the
Lungs is SSSSSSS.
Just like a snake!

So, now we're going to breathe in Courage, and
breathe out Sadness using the SSSSSS sound.
Remember to breathe out the dark smoke and let it go into the Earth.

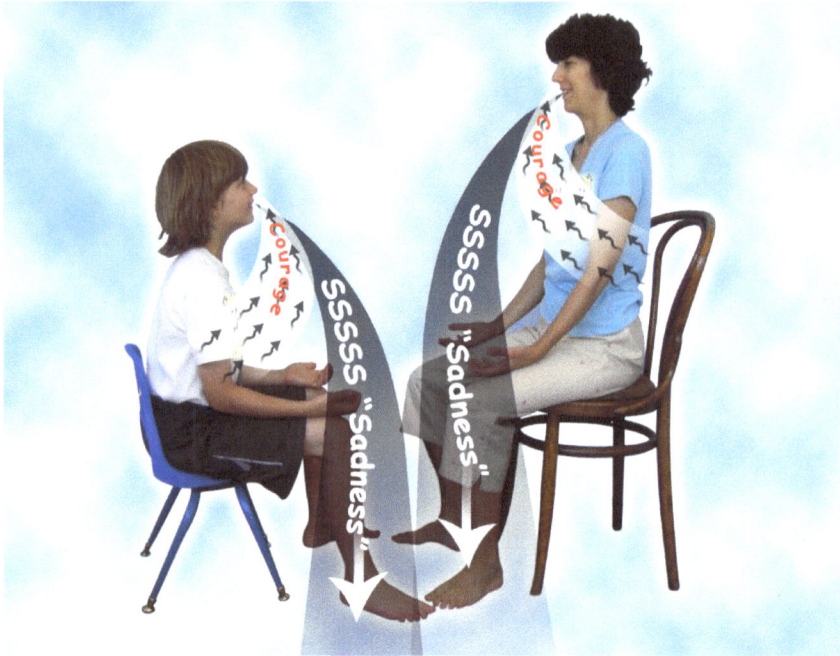

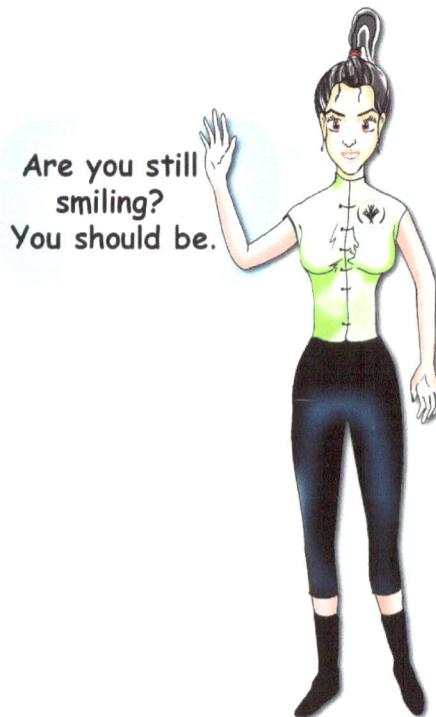

Are you still
smiling?
You should be.

I'M A CHI KID

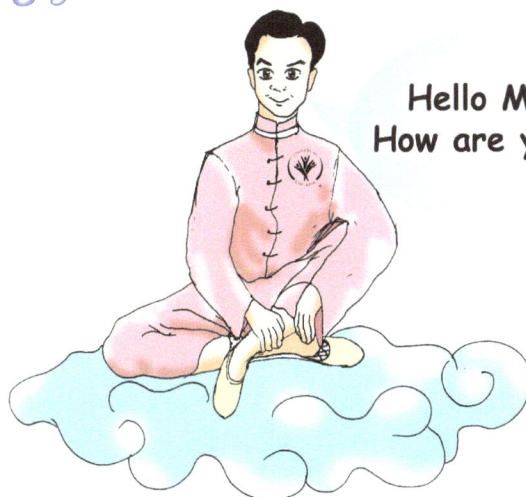

Hello Mr. Tiger.
How are you today?

Before I go, let me introduce you to my special friend.
This friend is like a guardian angel for your Lungs.
Ladies and gentlemen, The White Tiger!

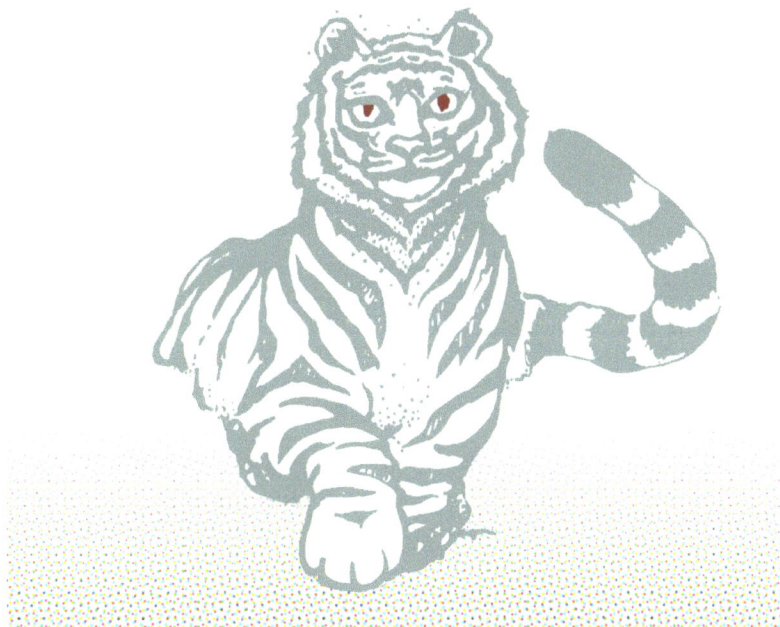

In the Taoist way, we believe there are special animals
to protect us from harm. When you smile to your shiny White Lungs,
smile to the White Tiger too!

Now let's put it all to gether.
Sit on a chair with your feet on the floor and SMILE.
FEEL YOUR LUNGS and SMILE TO YOUR LUNGS.
See your White Lungs smile back.
BREATHE IN THE FEELING OF COURAGE and fill
your Lungs with the White color.
BREATHE OUT SADNESS USING THE SSSS SOUND.
Let the dark smoke leave from your mouth and sink
into the earth. The Earth will use it to grow
something beautiful.

SAY"HELLO" TO THE WHITE TIGER that
protects your Lungs.
Smile one more time and FEEL THE COURAGE
flowing from your Lungs.

Try to do this 3 times in a row!

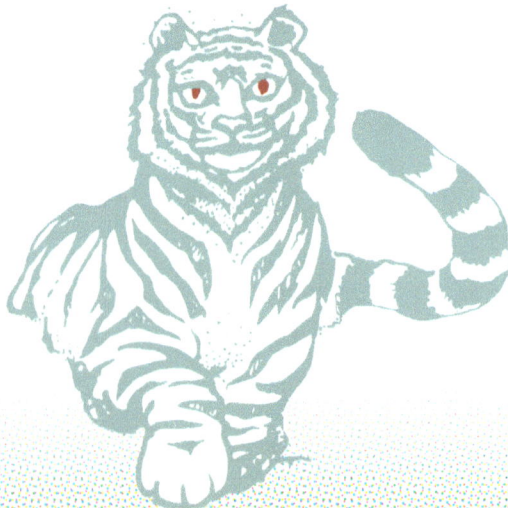

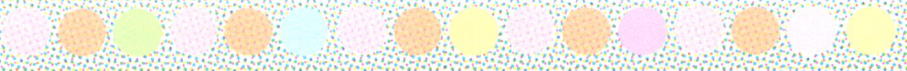

It is always important to take a little time to rest after we smile
to our Lungs. Just take one or two minutes and
think of what a brave person you are.

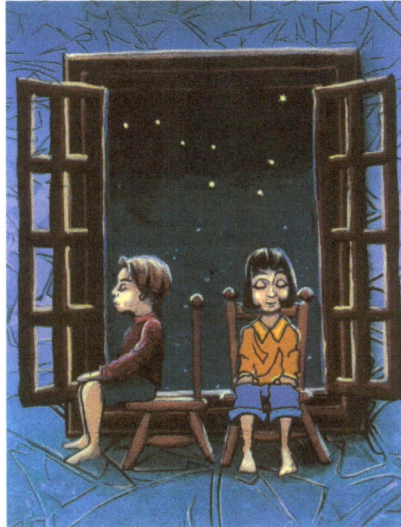

Remember, YOU are a very special person!

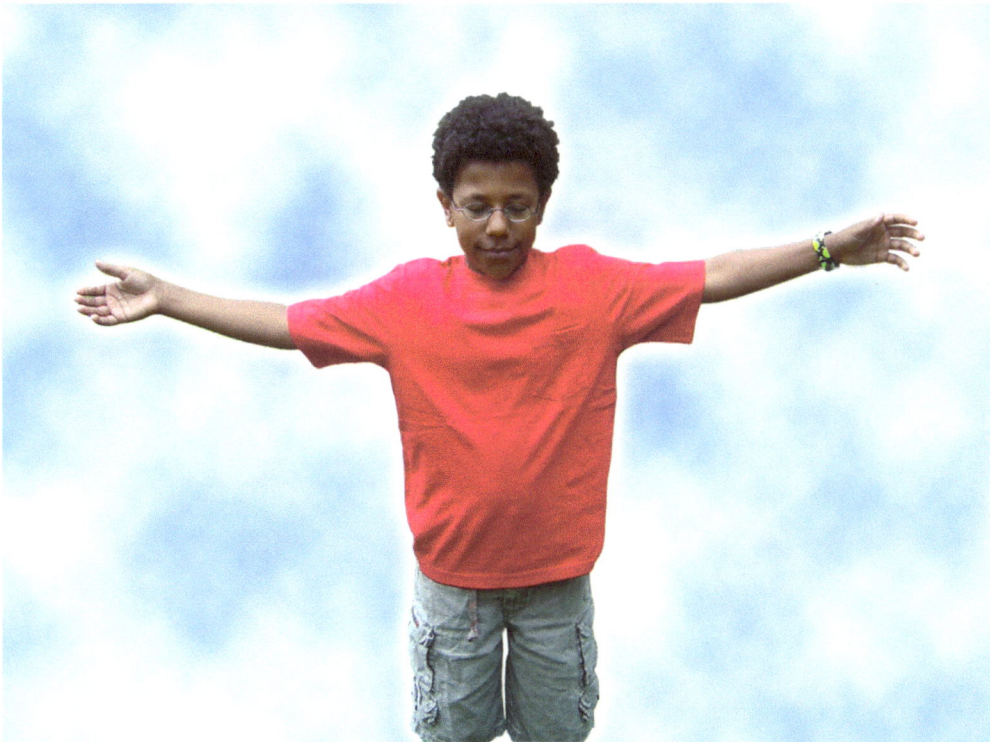

Chapter 3
Kidneys Sound

Recommended for ages 5-7
I can Smile to my Kidneys

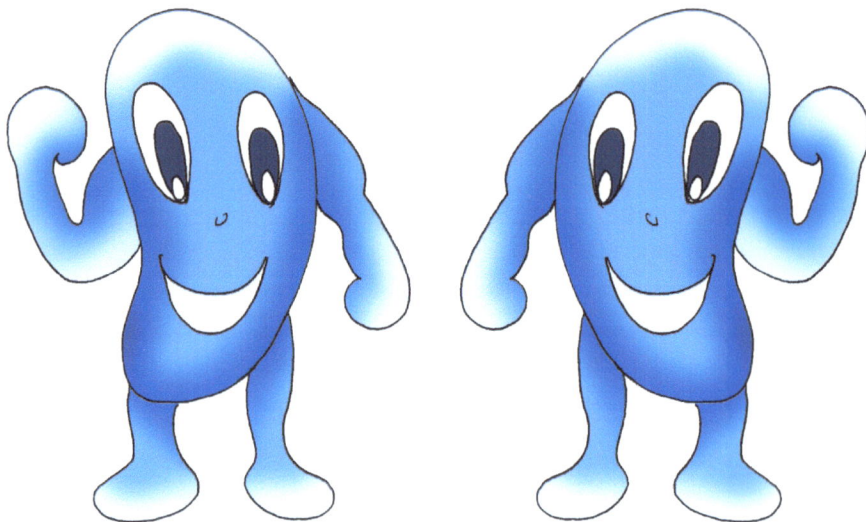

Inner Smile & Sounds That Heal

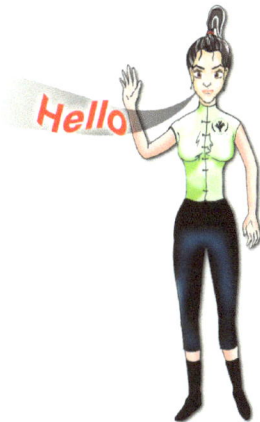

Welcome to Chi Kids "I Can Smile To My Kidneys" Level I.
My name is Sarina.
I am very excited to share this magic formula with you.
My teacher, Master Smile, taught me how to Smile to my Kidneys a long time ago
and now I am going to share with you.
Once you learn this secret, be sure to teach it to someone else!
Remember, we call this special magic, Chi Kung. Chi is energy and Kung is work, so
Chi Kung means "energy work" in Chinese.

This chapter will teach you where your Kidneys are, how to Smile to them,
how to talk to them and how to make yourself feel happier just by
thinking happy thoughts.

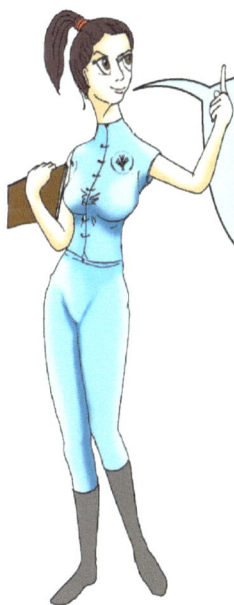

When a person uses their mind to change something inside or outside of their body, we call it MEDITATION.
Ask your grown-up to tell you more.

I'M A CHI KID

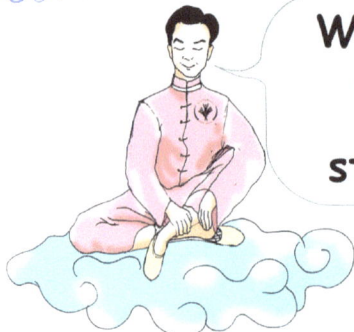

We are going to take a magical
adventure inside our body.
All you need to get
started is a great big smile.

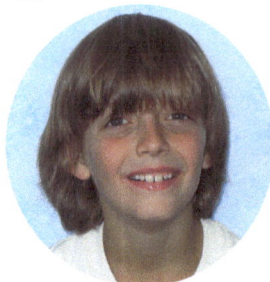

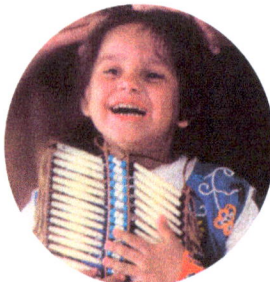

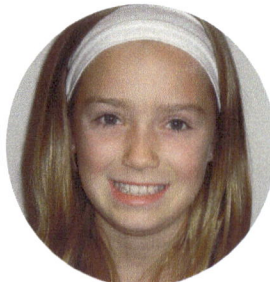

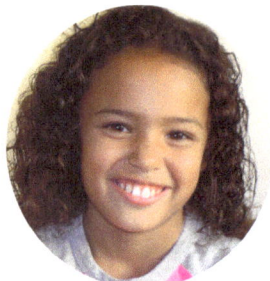

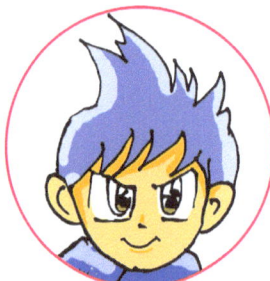

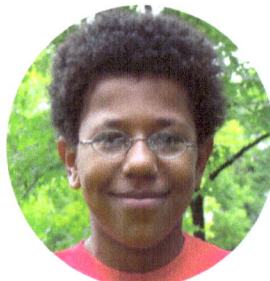

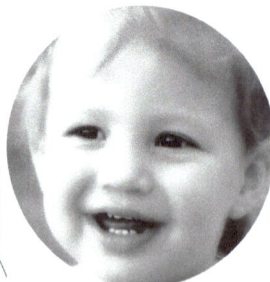

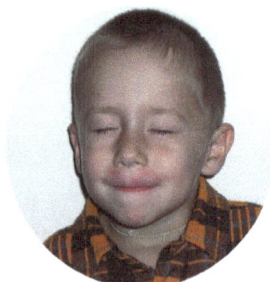

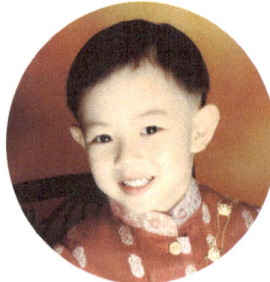

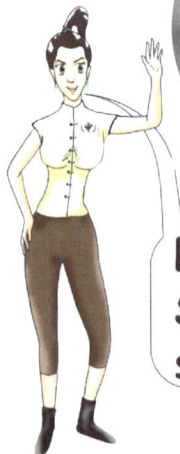

Look everyone. Its Master Smile!
Smile real big and you will see him
smile back!

You have a body.

You are the only person in the whole world born with your body.

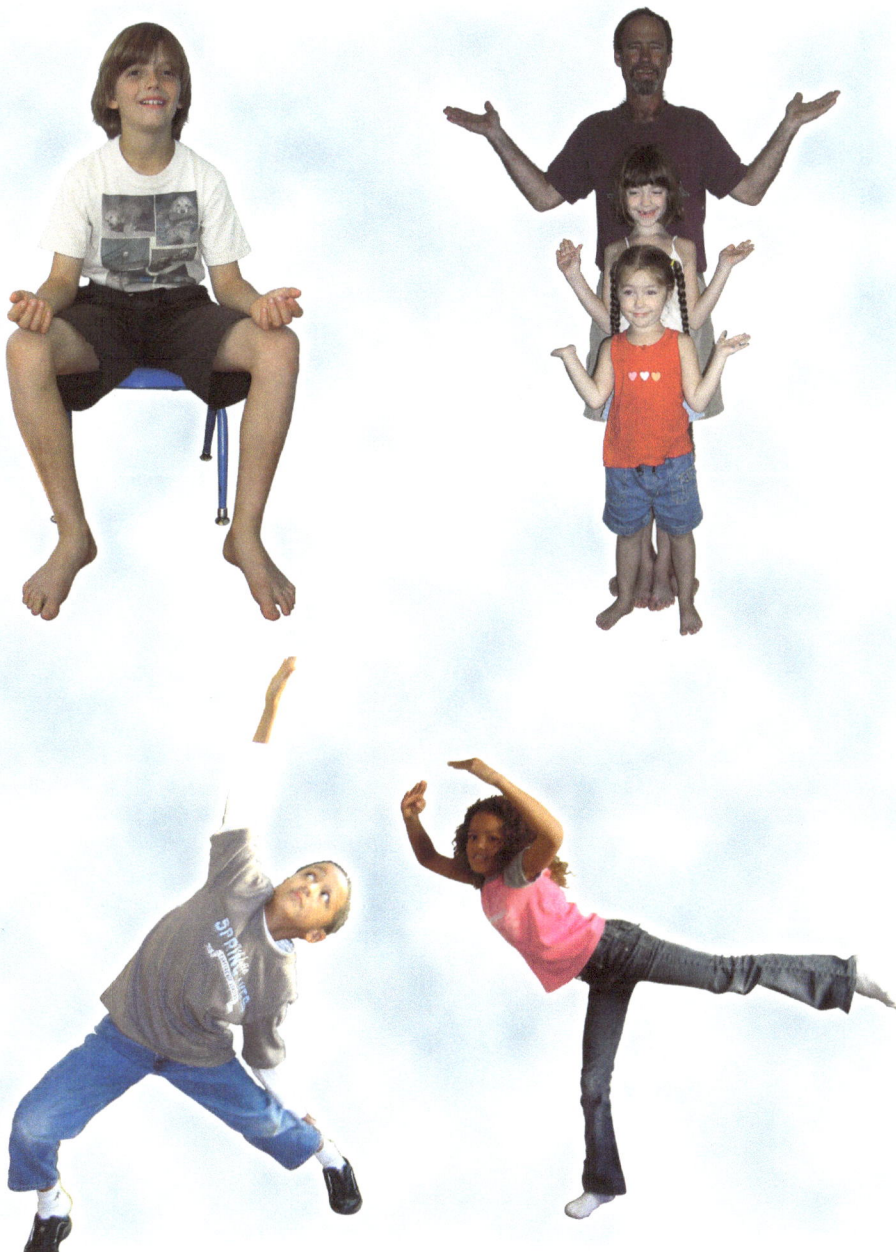

That makes you very special.

Your body has many parts.
Some parts are outside.

Outside

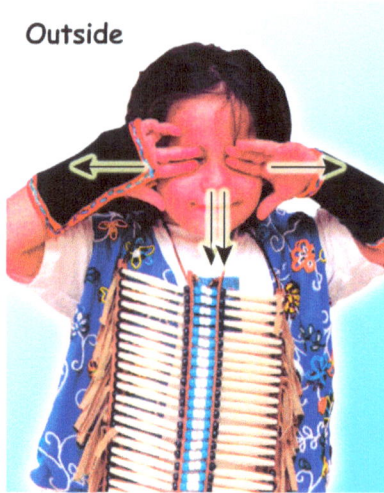

Some parts are inside.

Inside

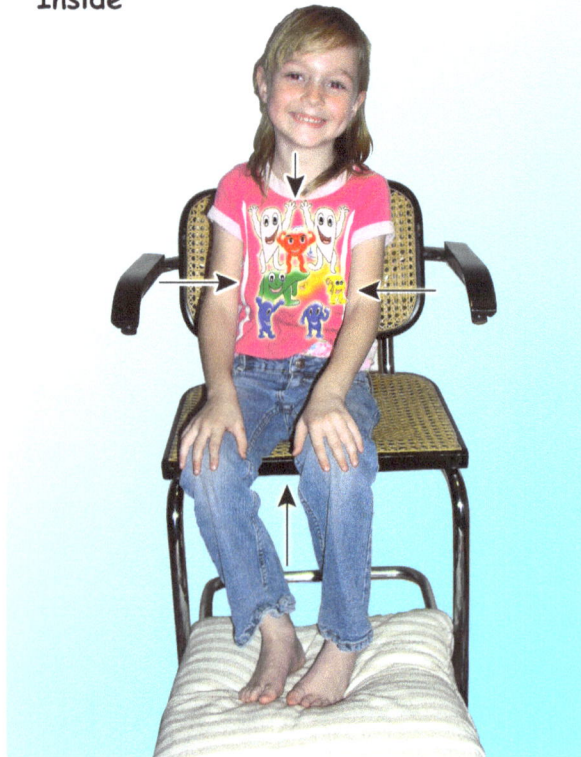

Today we will learn how to talk to your Kidneys.
And your Kidneys will learn to talk to you!!!!

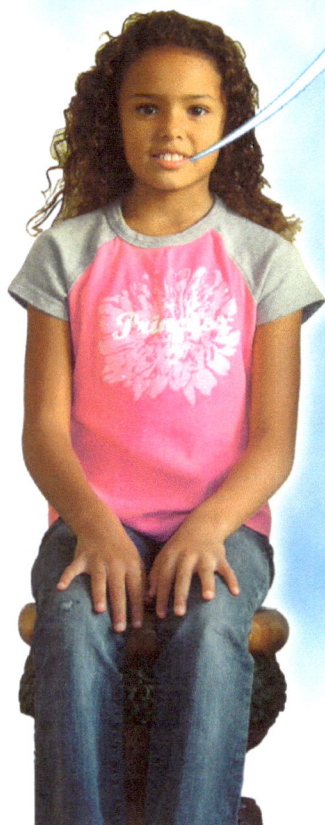
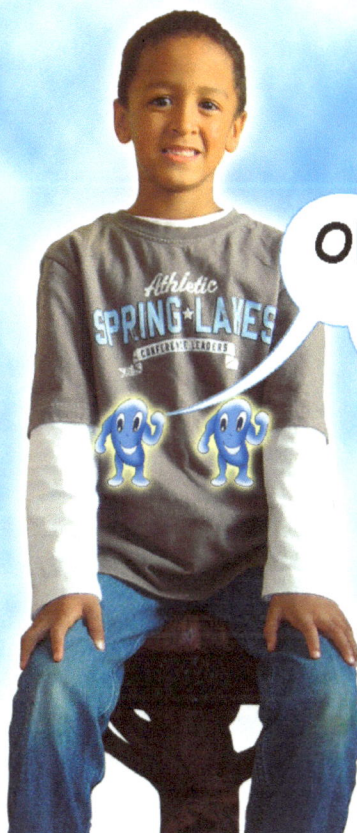

Begin by sitting on a chair with your feet on the ground.
Then, be quiet and feel where your Kidneys are.
Here is a picture to help you find them.
Reach your hands behind your back and let your fingertips
meet in the middle one your spine.
Look at the picture here and move your hands around
until you've found the right spots.

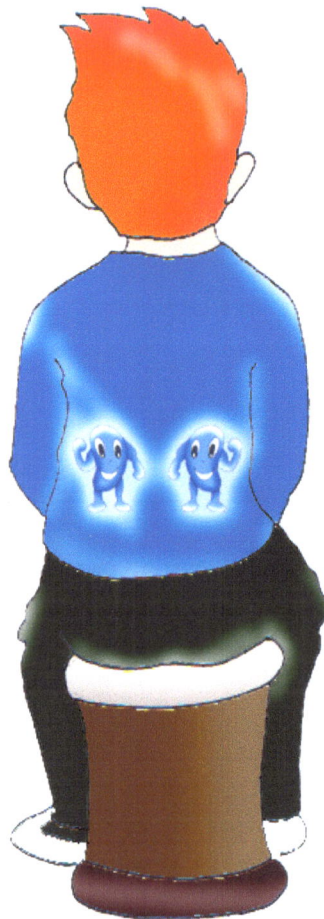

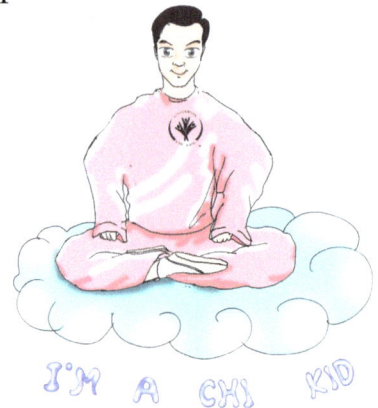

I'M A CHI KID

Remember, your Kidneys are underneath your bottom ribs in the back.
Be sure to ask your grown up what your Kidneys do to keep your body
clean and healthy.

Here is the most important step.
Put a big Smile on your face!

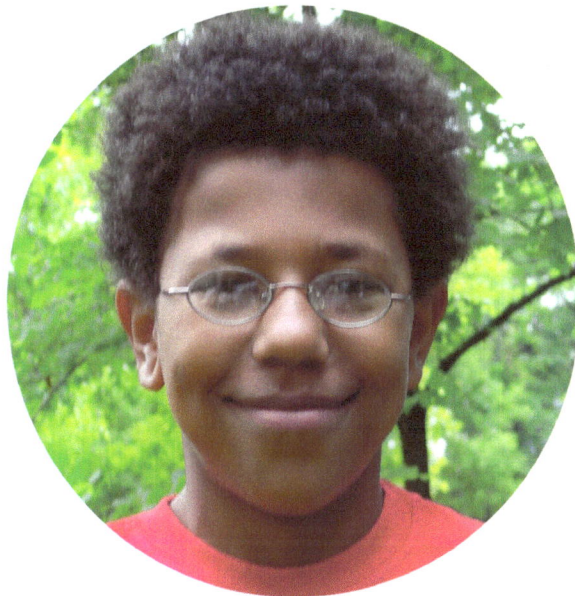

Take a deep breath and Smile to your Kidneys.
Let your Kidneys Smile back!
Be sure to breathe out when you're finished!!

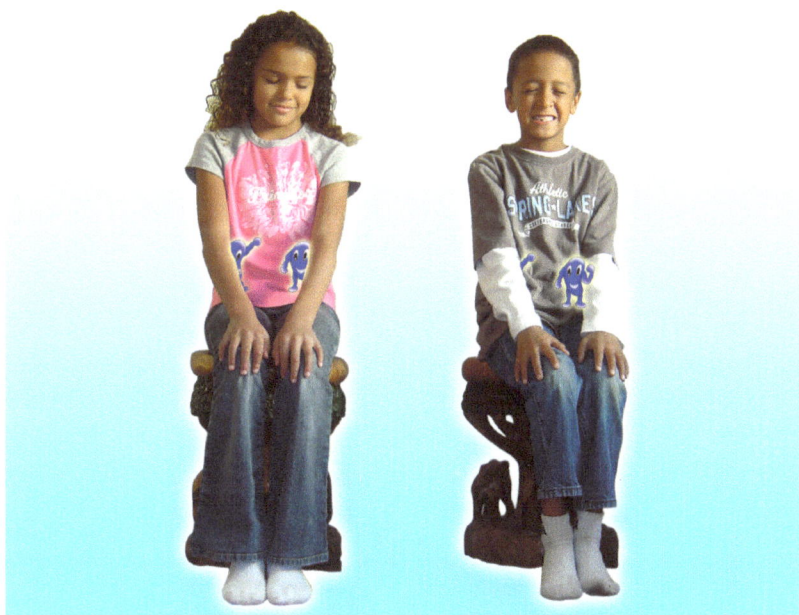

Imagine your Kidneys as a beautiful Blue color.

Next, close your eyes, Smile to your Kidneys and
breathe in the feeling of Gentleness.

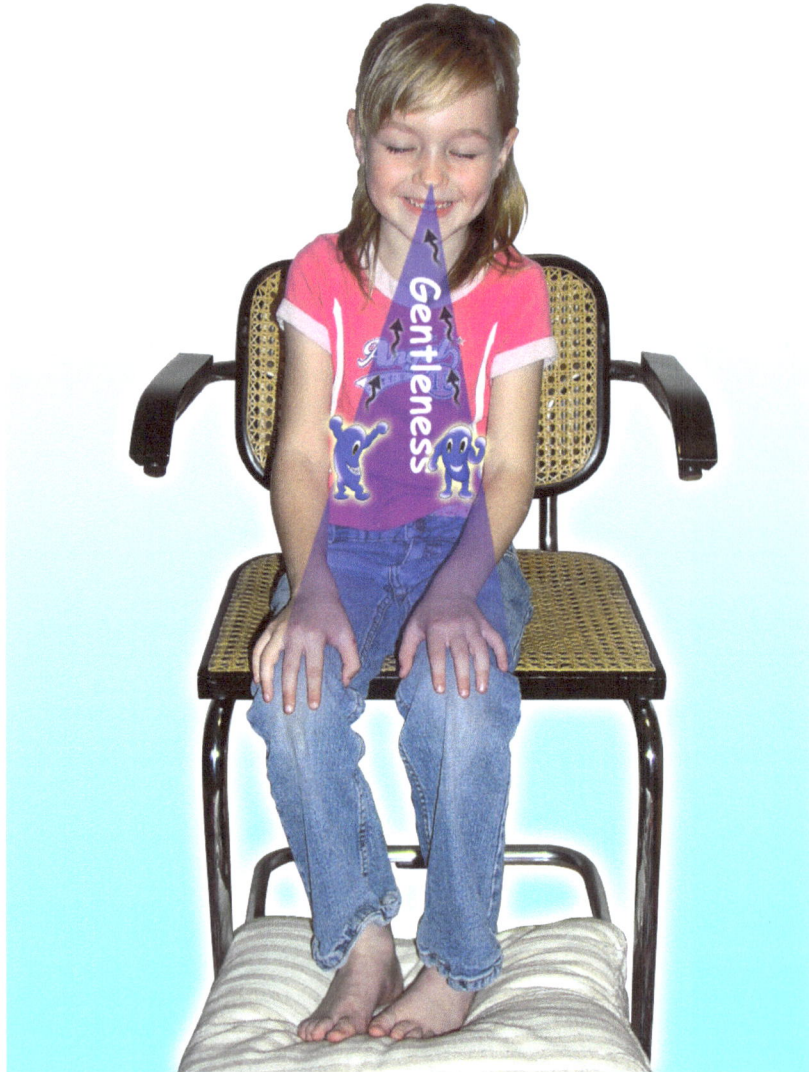

Fill your beautiful Blue Kidneys with the Blue color of Gentleness by
breathing in the beautiful cool Blue mist of Gentleness.

43

Breathe out the feeling of Fear
and being afraid.
See a dark smoke leave through your
mouth and drop down into the earth.

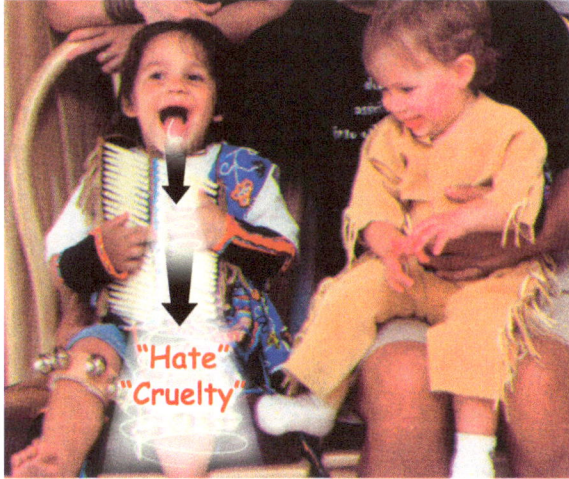

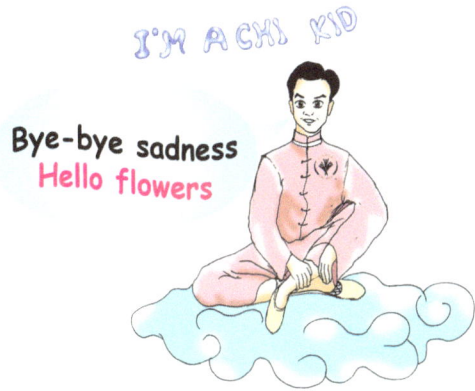

I'M A CHI KID

Bye-bye sadness
Hello flowers

"Hate"
"Cruelty"

The Earth will take your Fear and
use it to grow beautiful things like
flowers, tree's.

We call that transformation.
Can you say transformation?

Smile again to your beautiful,
Gentle, Blue Kidneys.

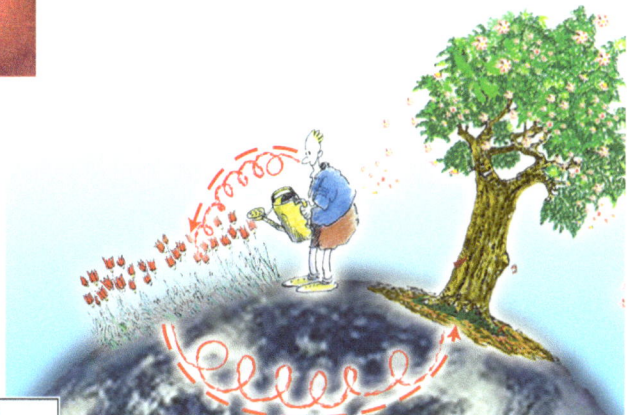

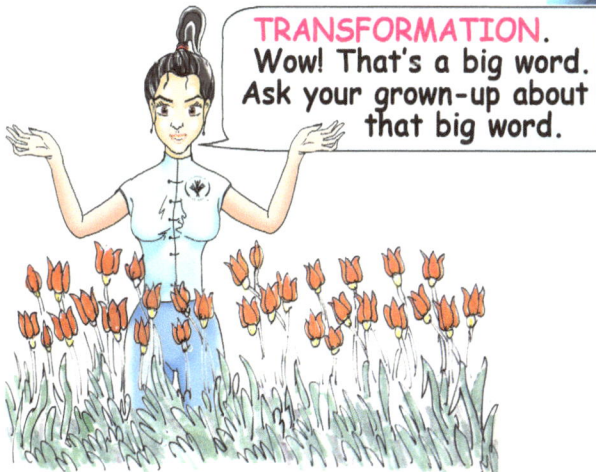

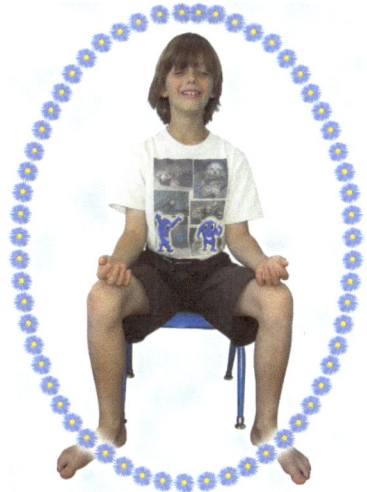

TRANSFORMATION.
Wow! That's a big word.
Ask your grown-up about
that big word.

44

Lets try it again. This time, we're going to speak
to our Kidneys out loud! The special healing
sound of the Kidneys is CHOOOO.

We make this sound with no voice. It's sort of like
blowing out the candles on a birthday cake.

Can you say CHOOOO?

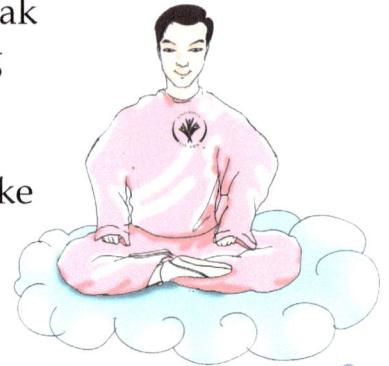

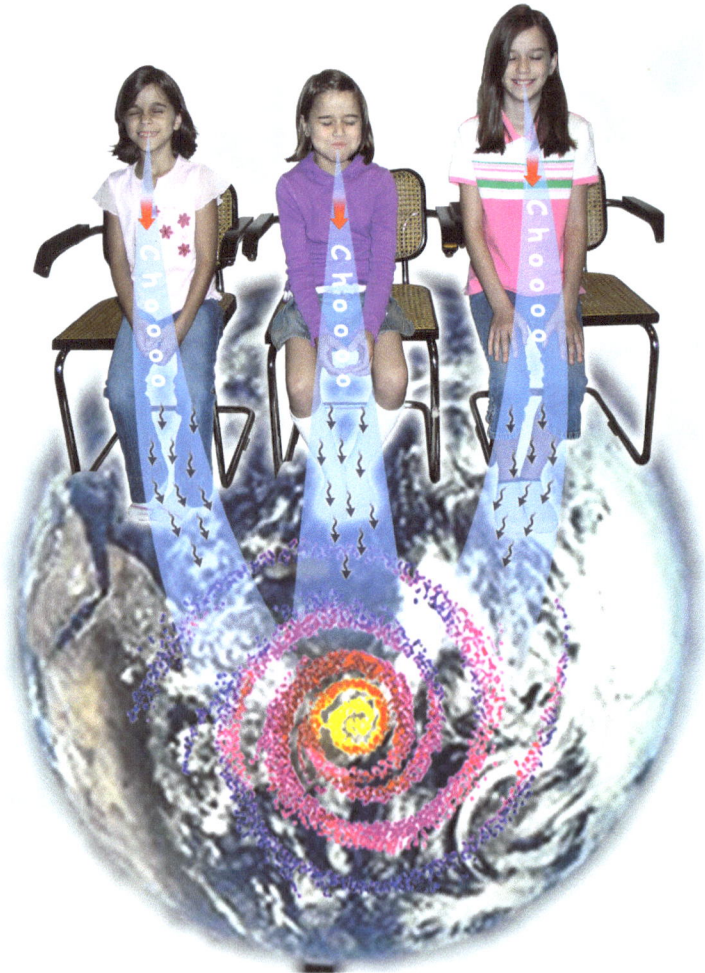

So, now we're going to breathe in Gentleness and breathe out Fear using
the CHOOOO sound.

Remember to breathe out the dark smoke and let it go into the Earth.
Let all the Fear out of your Kidneys when you breathe out and
let the feeling of Gentleness fill them up.

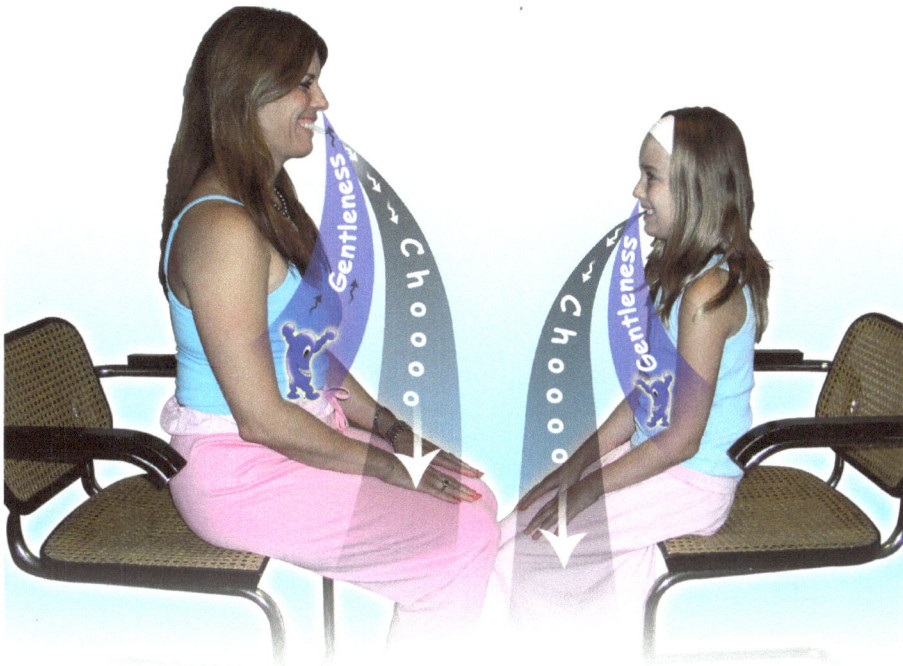

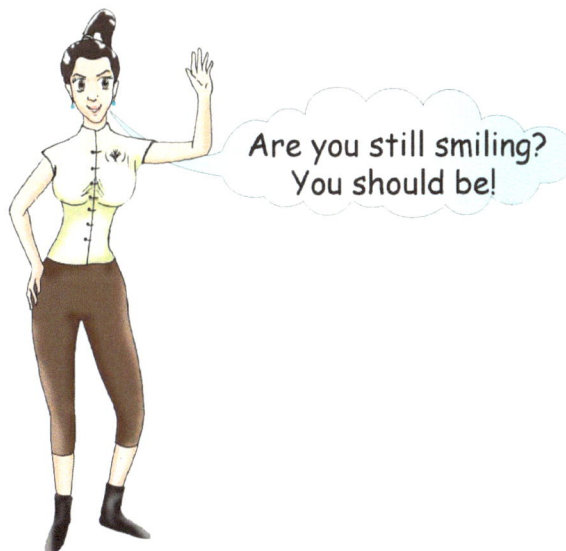

Look who's here! It's the Blue Turtle!
The Blue turtle is like a guardian angel for your Kidneys.

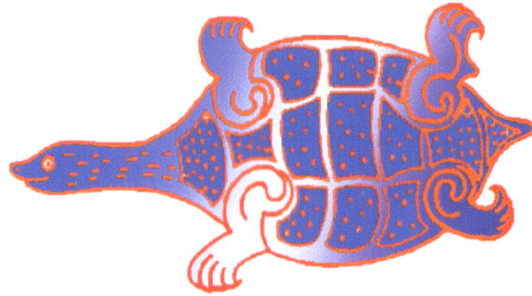

Ladies and gentlemen, The Blue Turtle! In the Taoist way, we believe there are special animals to protect us from harm. When you Smile to your beautiful Blue Kidneys, Smile to the Blue Turtle too!

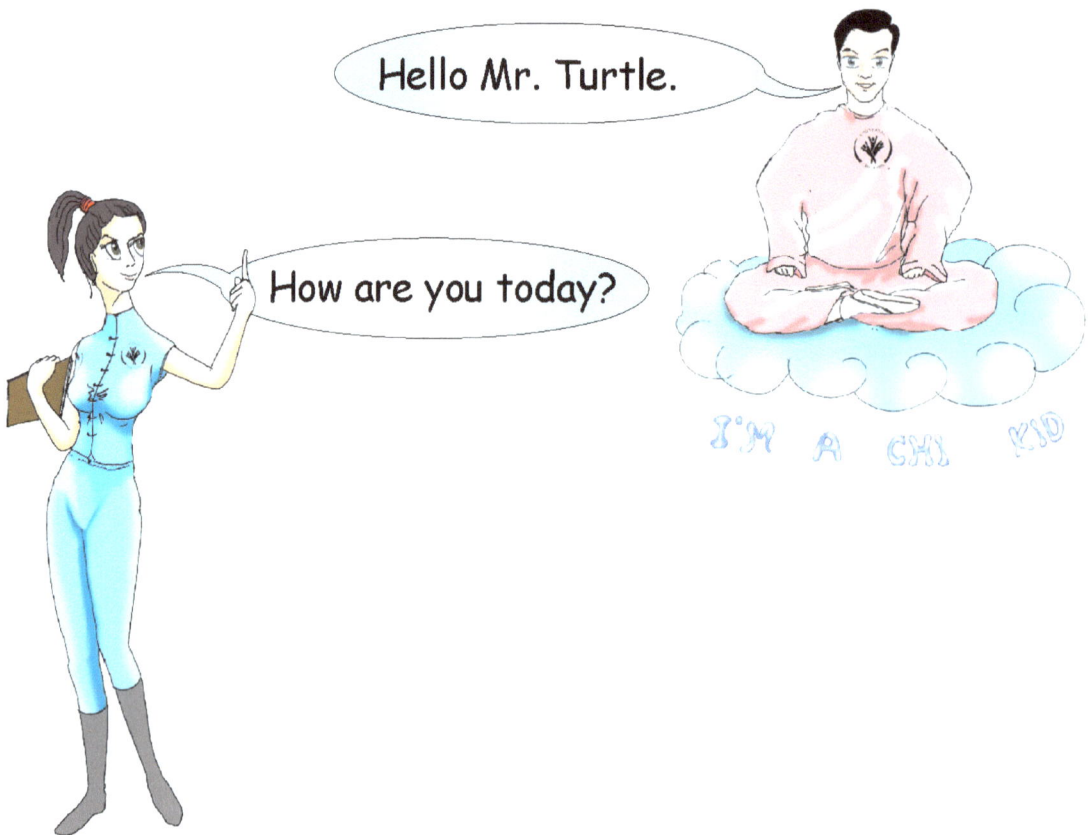

Hello Mr. Turtle.

How are you today?

47

Now, let's put it all together.
Sit on a chair with your feet on the floor and Smile.
Feel your Kidneys and Smile to your Kidneys.
See your Blue Kidneys Smile back.
Breathe in the feeling of gentleness and fill your Kidneys
with the Blue color.
Breathe out fear using the CHOOO sound.
Let the dark smoke leave from your mouth and sink into the earth. The
Earth will use it to grow something beautiful.
Say "Hello" to the Blue Turtle that protects your Kidneys.
Smile one more time and feel the Gentleness
flowing from your Kidneys.

Try to do this 3 times in a row!

It is always important to take a little time to rest after we Smile to our
Kidneys. Just take one or two minutes and be very Gentle.

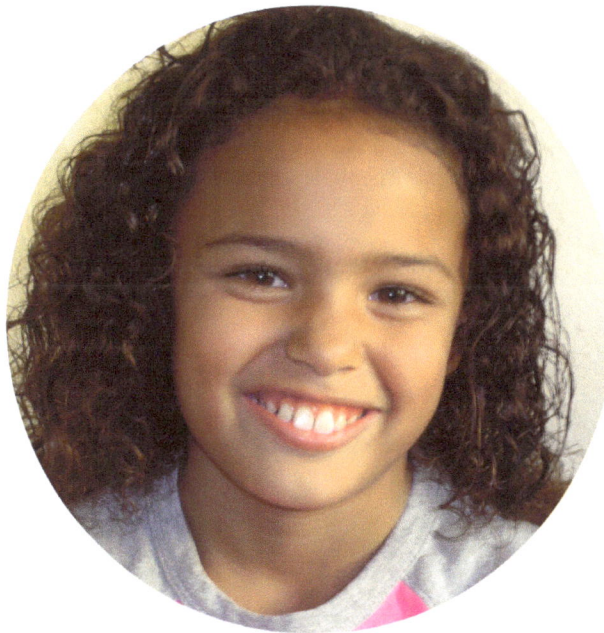

Remember, YOU are a very special person!

Chapter 4
Liver Sound

Recommended for ages 5-7
I can Smile to my Liver

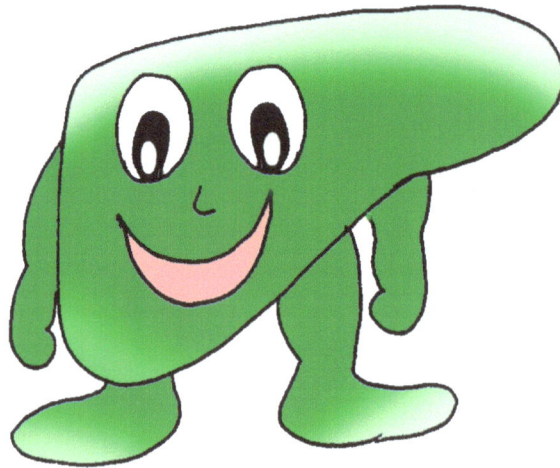

Inner Smile & Sounds That Heal

Hello

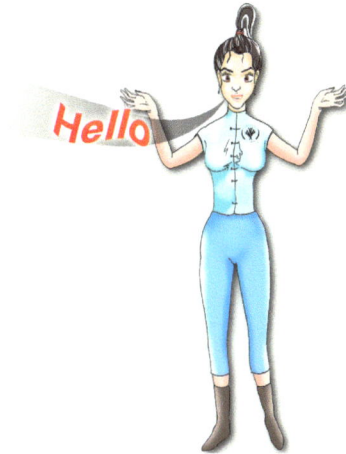

Welcome to Chi Kids "I Can Smile To My Liver" Level I.
My name is Sarina.
I am very excited to share this magic formula with you.
My teacher, Master Smile, taught me how to Smile to my Liver
a long time ago and now I am going to share with you.
Once you learn this secret, be sure to teach it to someone else!

Remember we call this special magic, Chi Kung.
Chi is energy and Kung is work, so Chi Kung means "energy work" in Chinese.
Do you know anyone who speaks Chinese?

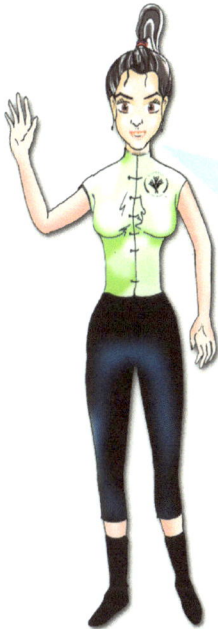

When a person uses their mind to change something inside or outside of their body, we call it MEDITATION. Ask your grown-up to tell you more.

This chapter will teach you
where your Liver is,
how to Smile to it, how to talk
to it and how to make yourself
feel happier just by thinking
happy thoughts.

You will learn to use your own energy to help
you feel better when you feel bad and be a happy,
healthy person.

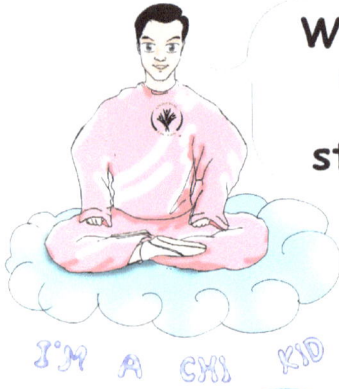

We are going to take a magical
adventure inside our body.
All you need to get
started is a great big smile.

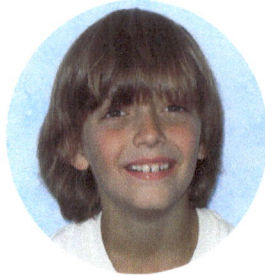

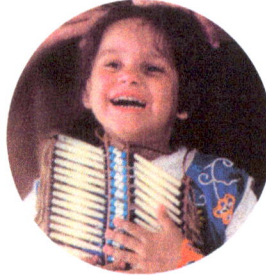

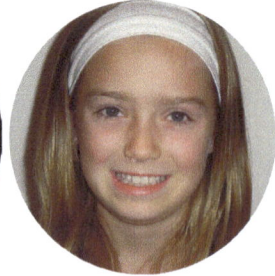

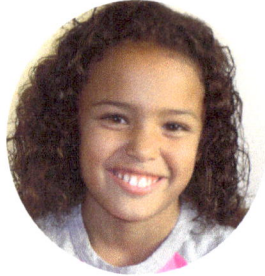

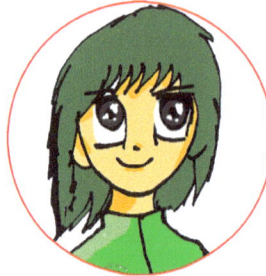

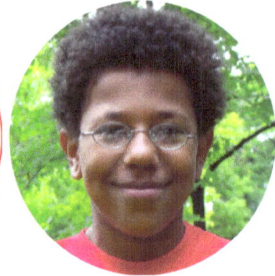

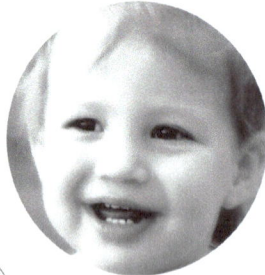

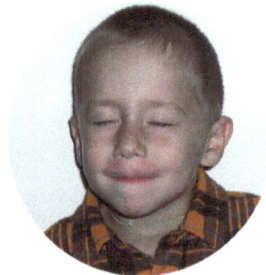

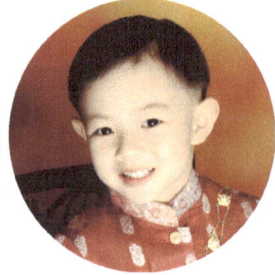

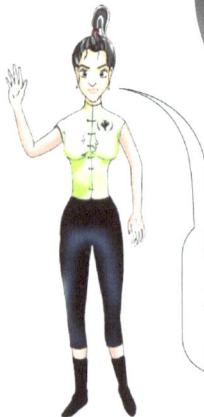

I'M A CHI KID

Look everyone. Its Master Smile!
Smile real big and you will see him
smile back!

53

You have a body.
You are the only person in the whole world born with your body.

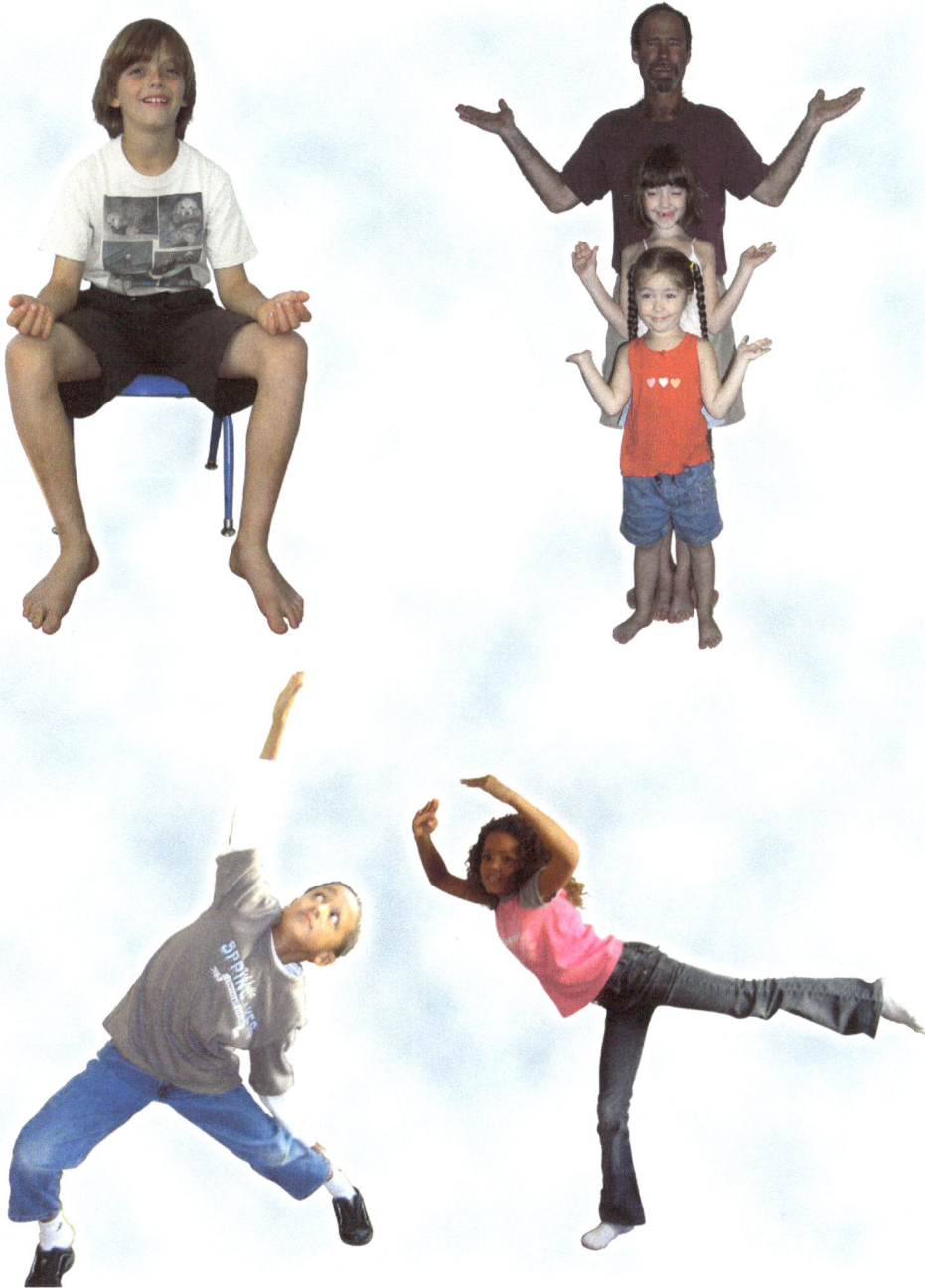

That makes you very special.

Your body has many parts.
Some parts are outside.

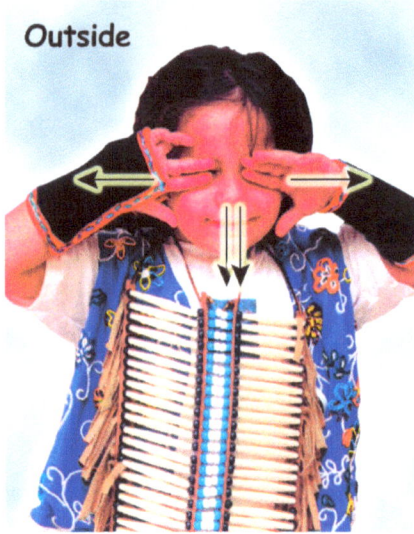

Outside

Some parts are inside.

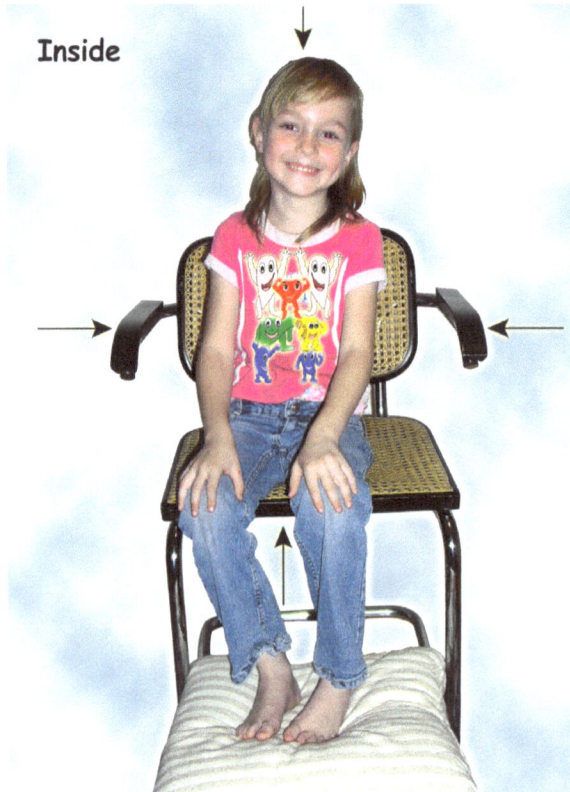

Inside

Today we will learn how to talk to your Liver.
And your Liver will learn to talk to you!!!!

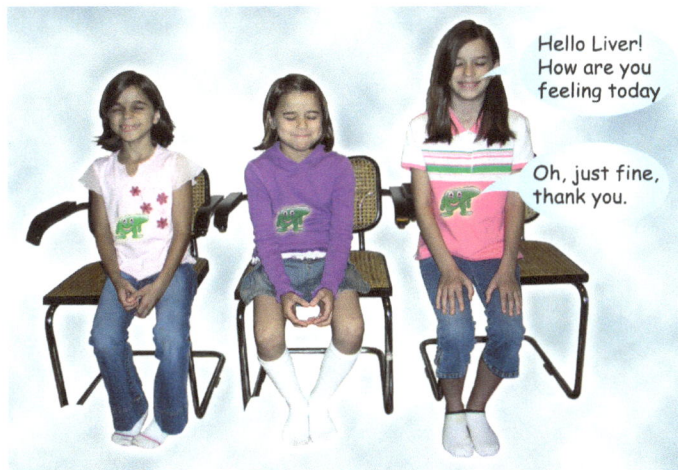

Begin by sitting on a chair with your feet on the ground.
Then, be quiet and feel where your Liver is.
Here is a picture to help you find it.

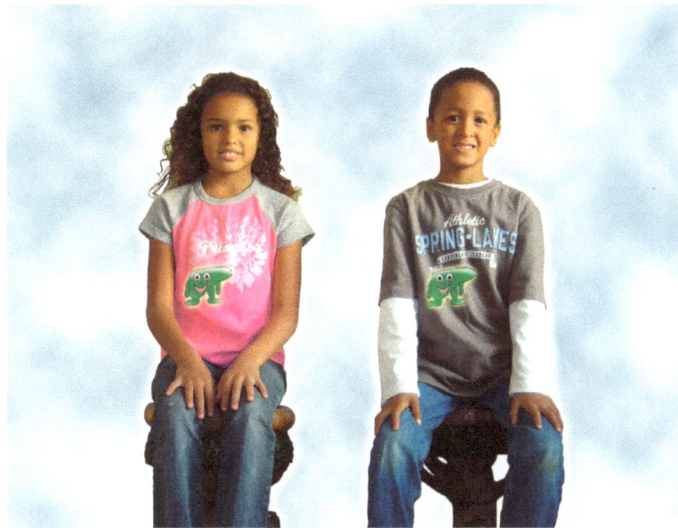

Look at the picture here and move your hands around
until you've found the right spot.
Remember, your Liver is underneath your ribs and stretches
from the front to the back of your rib cage.
Ask your grown up what the Liver does for you and your blood.

Here is the most important step.
Put a big Smile on your face!

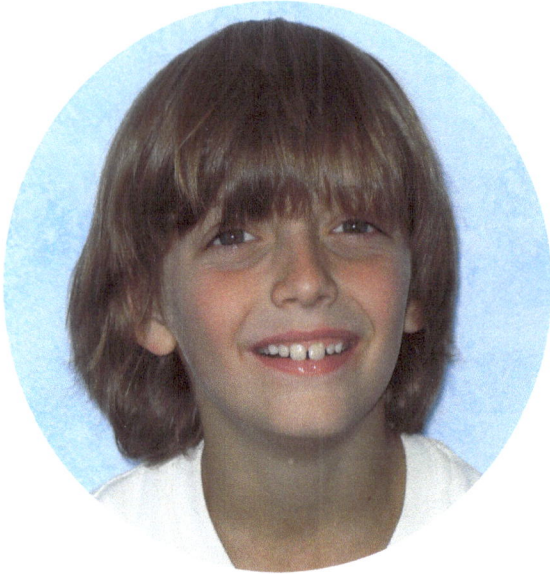

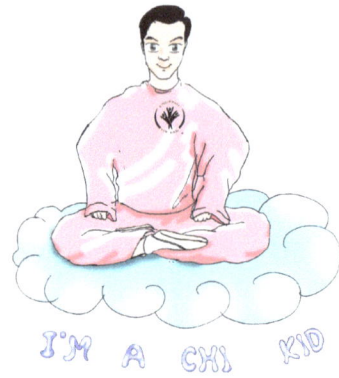

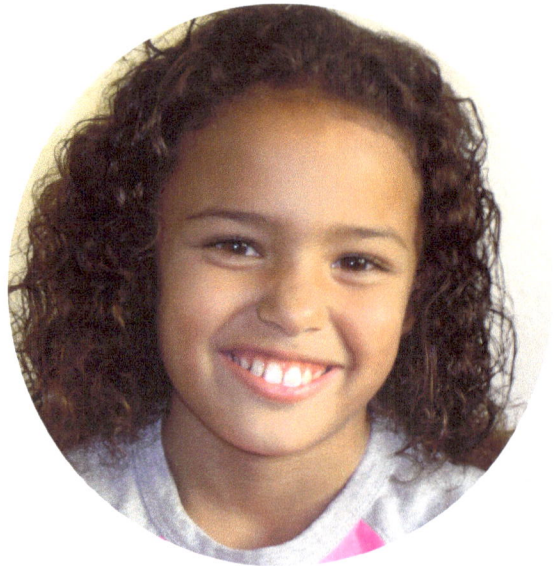

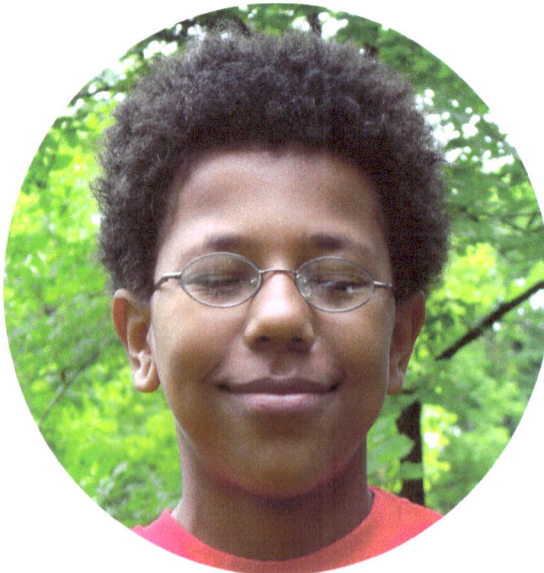

I'M A CHI KID

Take a deep breath and Smile to your Liver.
Let your Liver Smile back!
Be sure to breathe out when you're finished!!

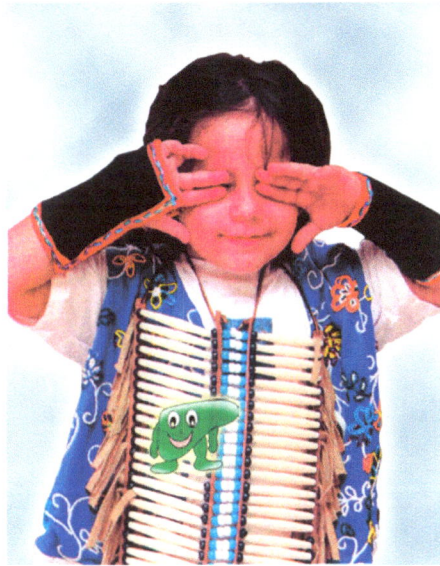

Imagine your Liver as a beautiful Green color.
Like an emerald with a light shining from inside.

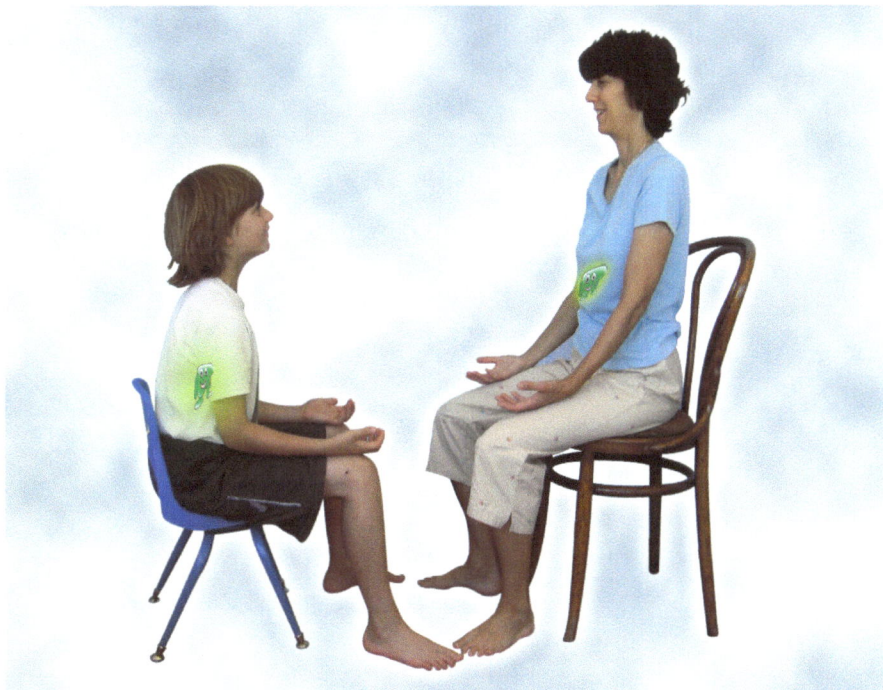

Close your eyes, Smile to your Liver and
breathe in the feeling of Kindness.

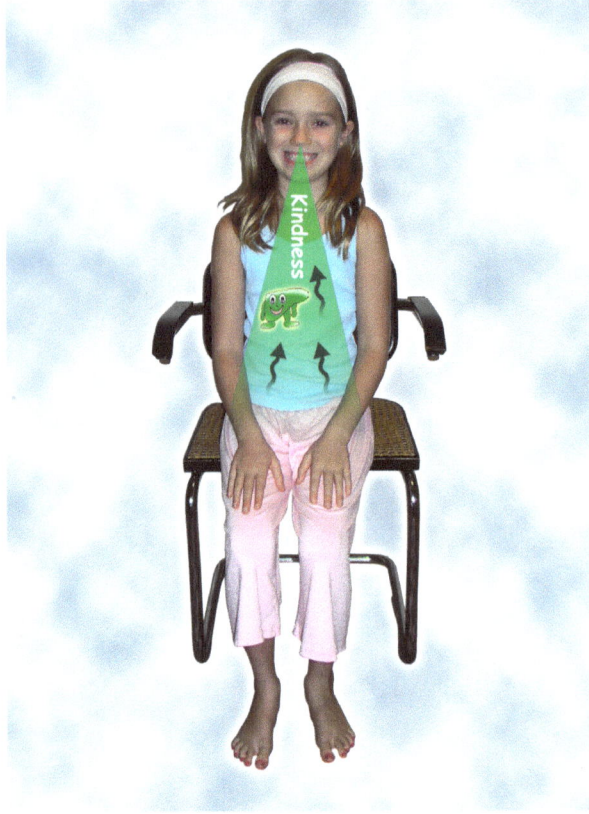

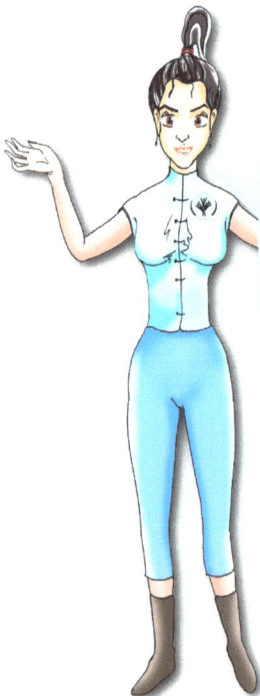

Breathe in the
beautiful cool Green
mist of Kindness and
see the Green color
fill your Liver.

59

Breathe out the feeling of Anger.
See a dark smoke leave through your mouth and
drop down into the earth.

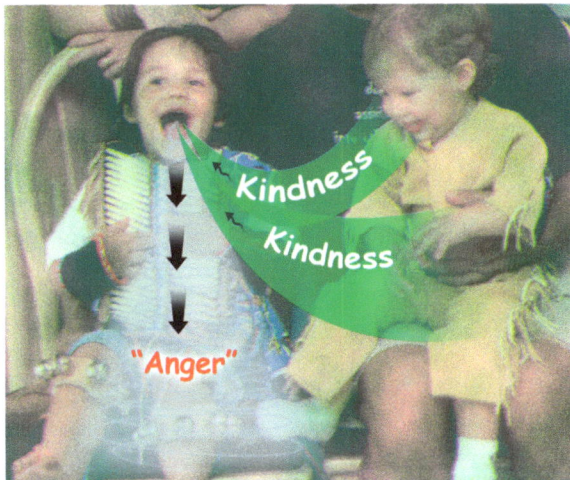

The Earth will take your garbage
and use it to grow
beautiful things, like flowers or trees.
We call that transformation.

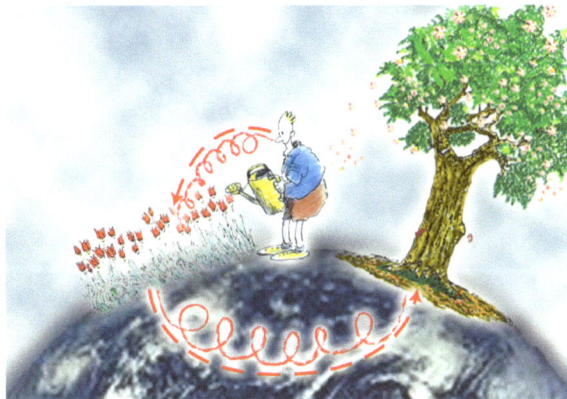

TRANSFORMATION.
Wow! That's a big word.
Ask your grown-up about
that big word.
Bye-bye Anger
Hello flowers

Smile to your
beautiful, Kind,
Green Liver.

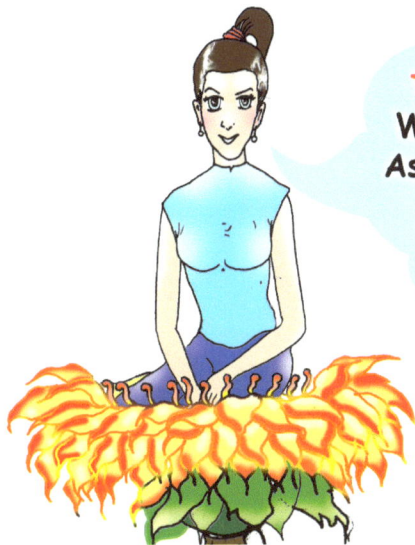

Lets try it again.
This time, we're going to speak to our
Liver out loud!
The special healing sound
of the Liver is Shhhh.

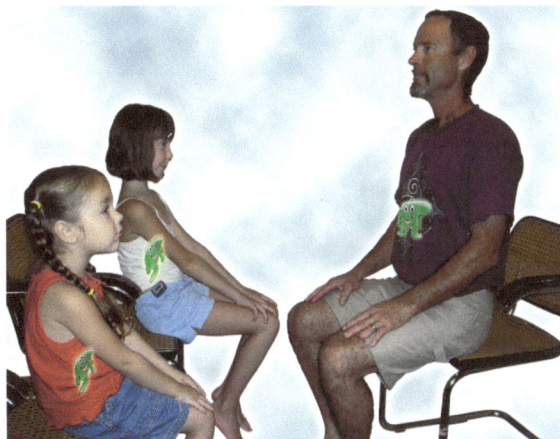

60

Can you say Shhhh?

So, now we're going to breathe in Kindness
and breathe out Anger
using the Shhhh sound. Remember to
breathe out the dark smoke and let it go
into the Earth. Let all the Anger out of your
Liver when you breathe out and let the feeling of Kindness fill it up.

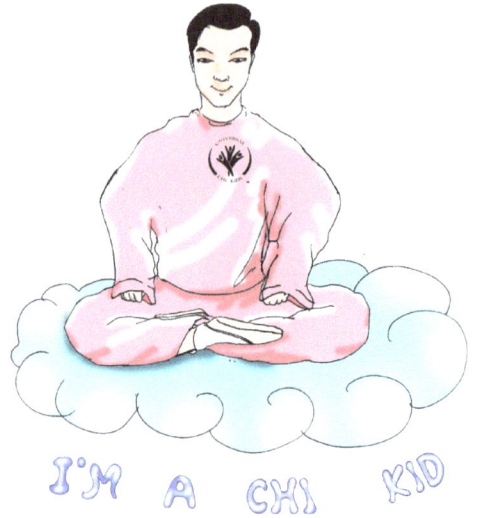

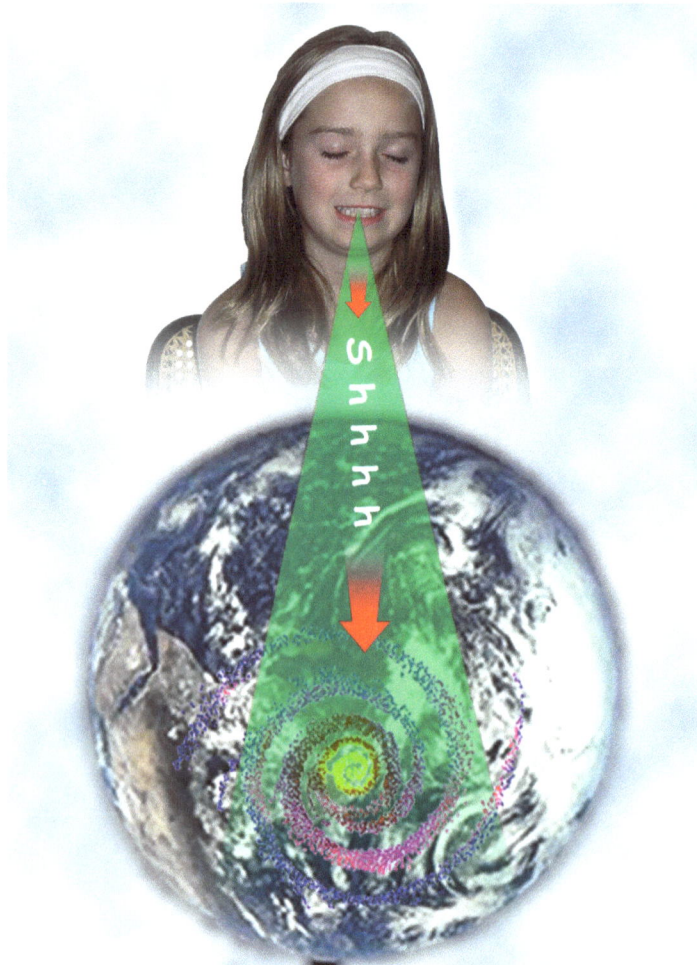

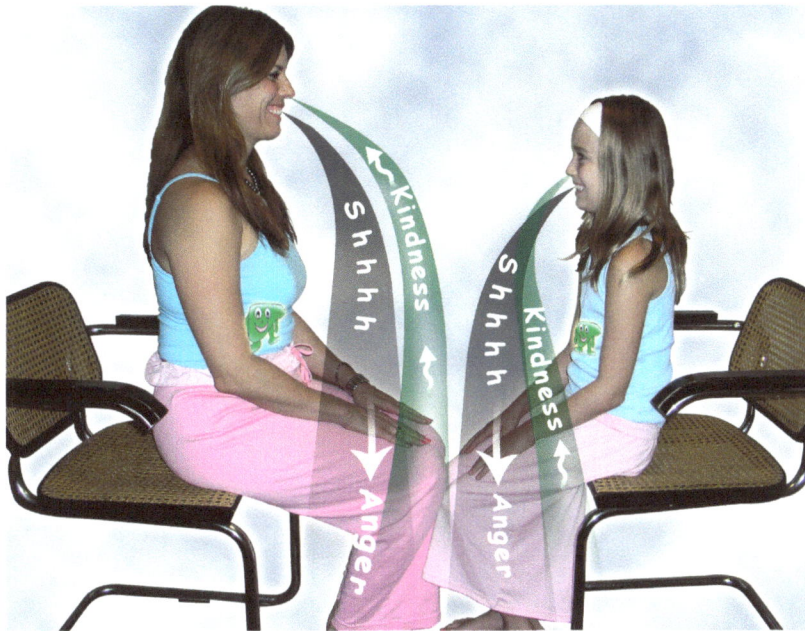

Look who's here!
This friend is like a guardian angel for your
Liver.
Ladies and gentlemen,
The Green Dragon!

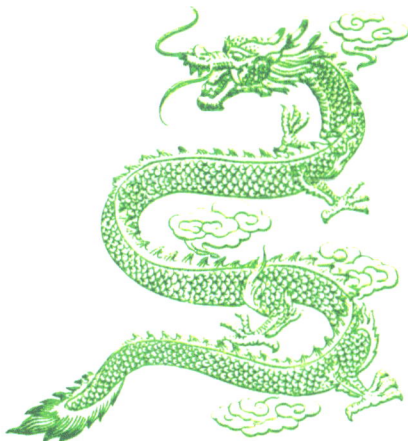

Are you still
smiling?
You should be!

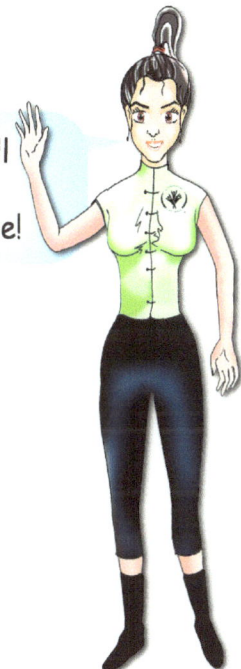

In the Taoist way, we believe there are special animals to protect us from
harm. When you Smile to your Green Liver,
Smile to the Green Dragon too!

I'M A CHI KID

Hello
Mr. Dragon

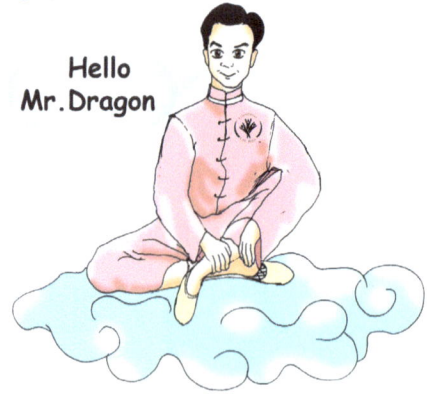

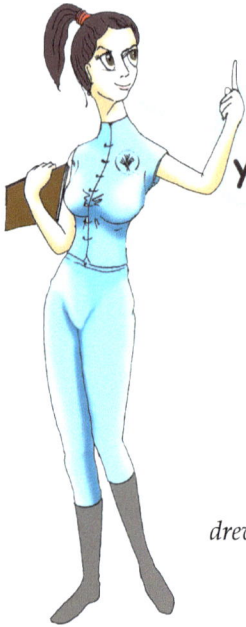

How are
you today?

My friend, Lucy,
drew this beautiful dragon!

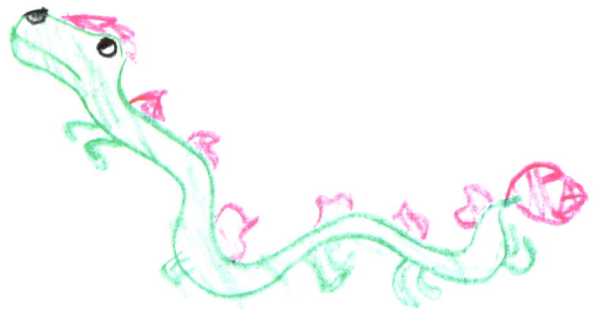

63

Let's put it all together!
Sit on a chair with your feet on the floor and Smile.
Feel your Liver and Smile to your Liver.
See your Green Liver smile back.
Breathe in the feeling of Kindness and fill your Liver
with the Green color.
Now, use the Shhhh sound and
breathe out anger and let the dark smoke leave from
your mouth and sink into the earth. The Earth will use
it to grow something beautiful.
Say "Hello" to the Green Dragon
that protects your Liver.
Smile one more time and feel the Kindness
flowing from your Liver.

Try to do this 3 times in a row!

It is always important to take a little time to rest after
we Smile to our Liver. Just take one or two minutes
and relax.   Can you think of a Kind person
in your life?

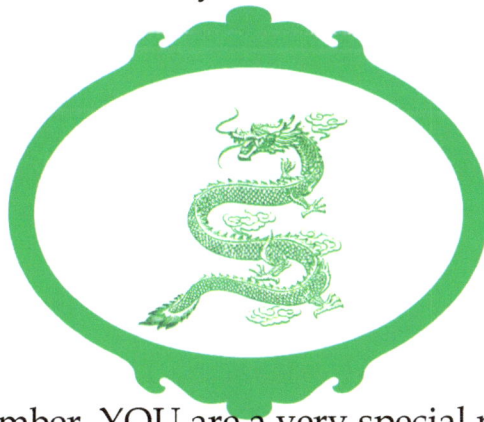

Remember, YOU are a very special person!

Chapter 5
Spleen & Pancreas Sound

Recommended for ages 5-7
I can Smile to my
Spleen & Pancreas

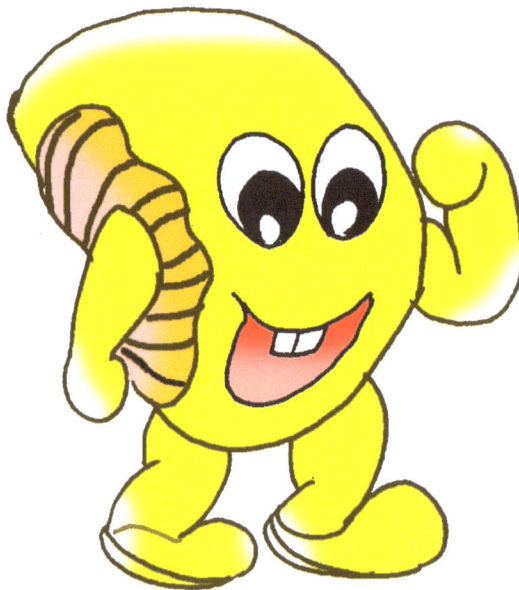

Inner Smile & Sounds That Heal

Hello

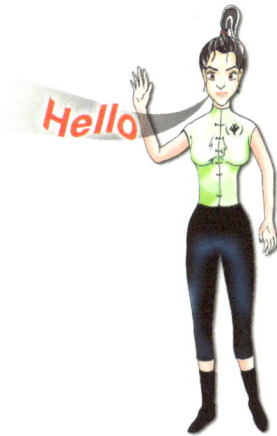

Welcome to Chi Kids "I Can Smile To My Spleen and Pancreas" Level I.
My name is Sarina. I am very excited to share this magic formula with you.
My teacher, Master Smile, taught me how to smile to my Spleen and Pancreas
a long time ago and now I am going to share with you. Once you learn this secret, be
sure to teach it to someone else!
Remember we call this special magic Chi Kung.
Chi is energy and Kung is work, so Chi Kung means "energy work" in Chinese.
Do you know anyone who speaks Chinese?

This chapter will teach you where your Spleen and Pancreas are,
how to Smile to them, how to talk to them and how to make
yourself feel happier just by thinking happy thoughts.

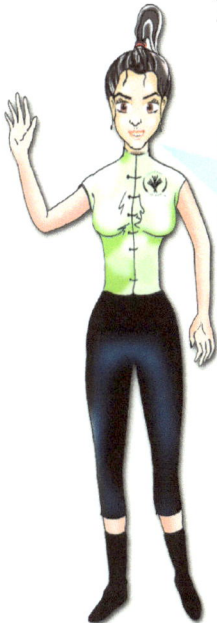

When a person uses their mind
to change something inside or
outside of their body, we call
it MEDITATION. Ask your
grown-up to tell you more.

You will learn to use your own energy to help
you feel better when you feel bad and be a happy,
healthy person.

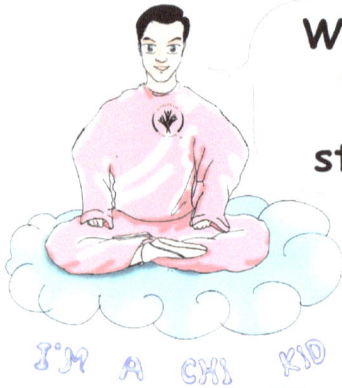

We are going to take a magical
adventure inside our body.
All you need to get
started is a great big smile.

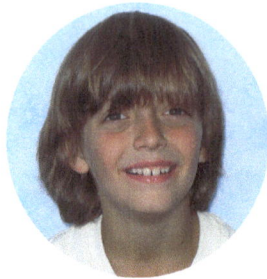

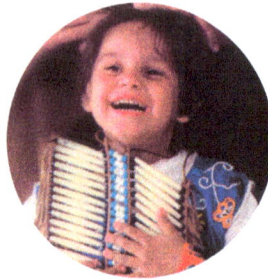

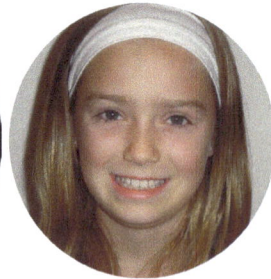

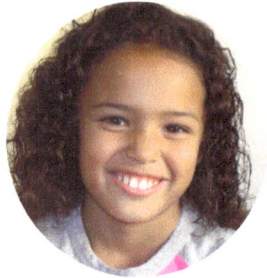

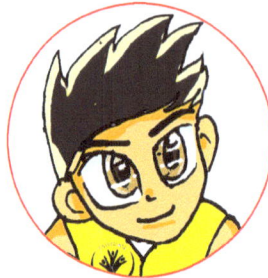

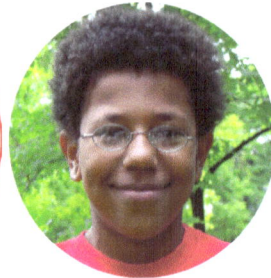

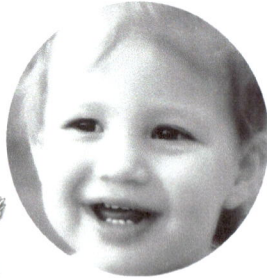

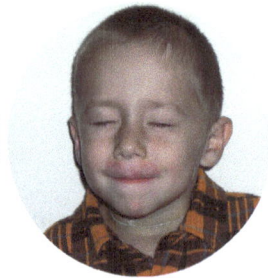

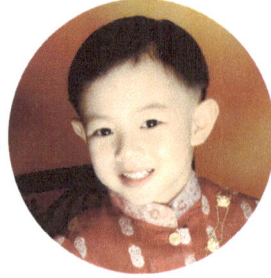

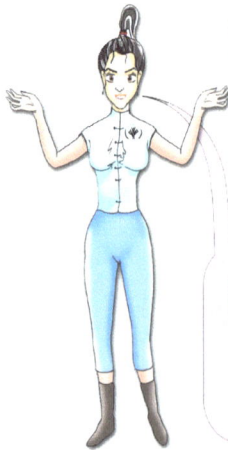

Look everyone! It's Master Smile!
Smile real big and you will see
him smile back!

You have a body.
You are the only person in the whole world born with your body.

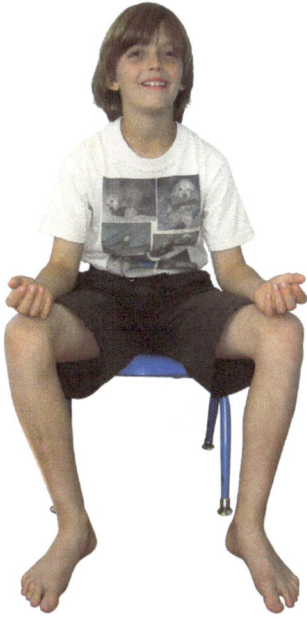

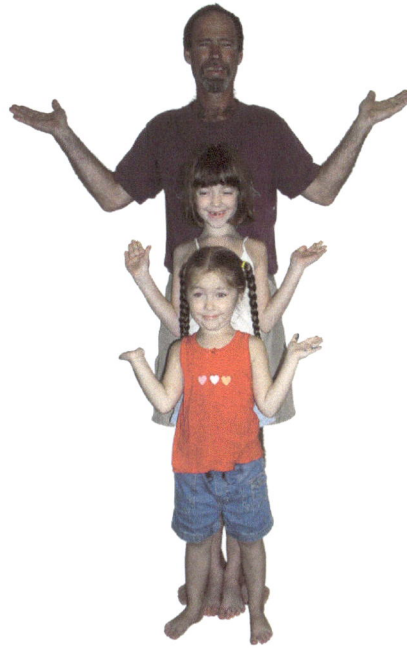

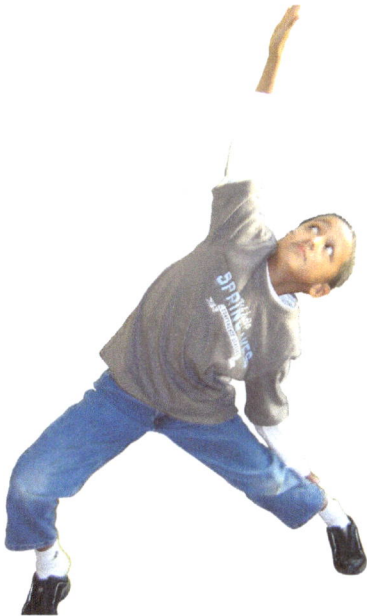

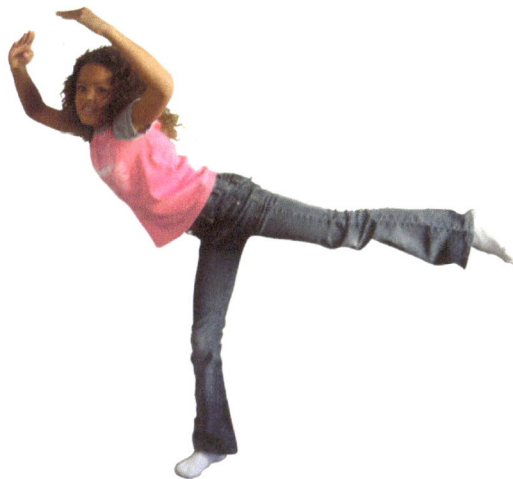

That makes you very special.

Your body has many parts.
Some parts are outside.   Some parts are inside.

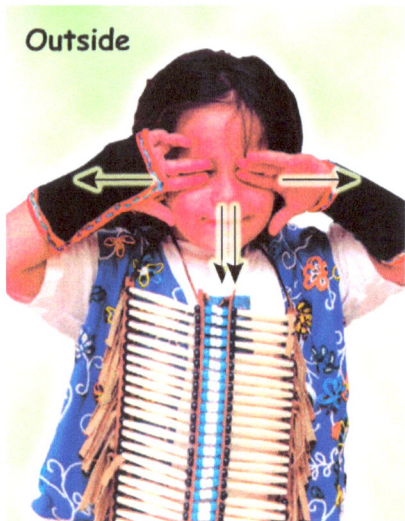

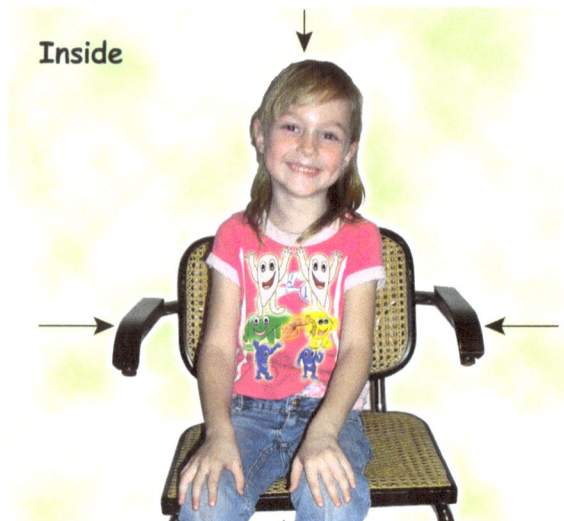

Outside

Inside

Today we will learn how to talk to your Spleen and Pancreas.
And they will learn to talk to you!!!!

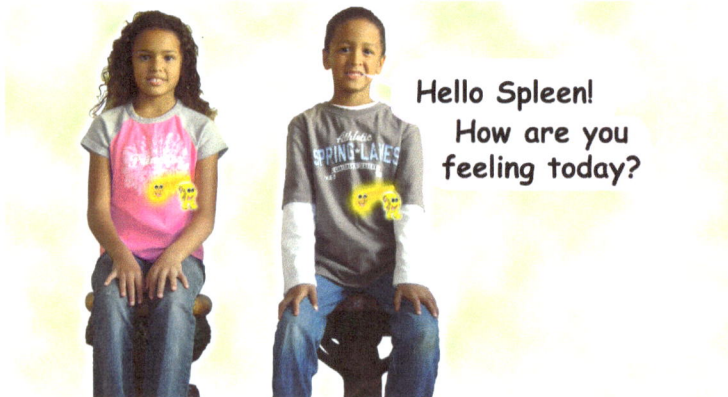

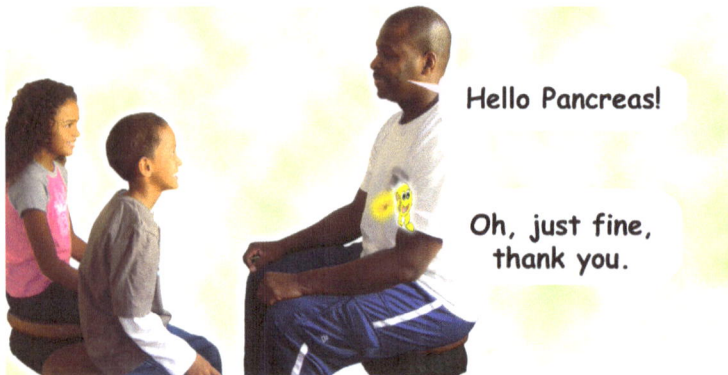

Hello Spleen!
How are you
feeling today?

Hello Pancreas!

Oh, just fine,
thank you.

We begin by sitting in a chair with our feet
on the ground and feeling where
our Spleen and Pancreas are.
If you are very quiet, you will feel them.

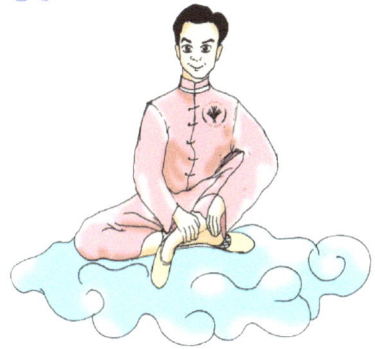

Ask your grown up for help finding the
Spleen on your left side and ask your grown up
what this organ does for your white "fighter"
blood cells.

Then, ask your grown up to help you find your
Pancreas right near your stomach. Have them explain to you what this
organ does for the sugar in your blood. Did you know there is sugar in
your blood?

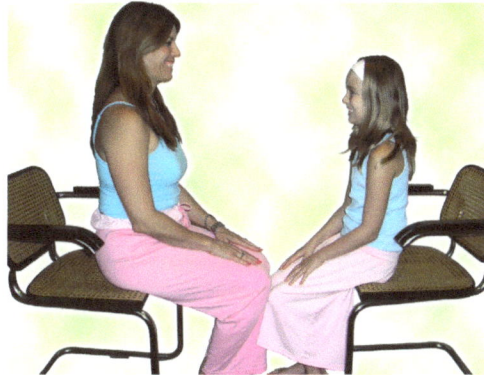

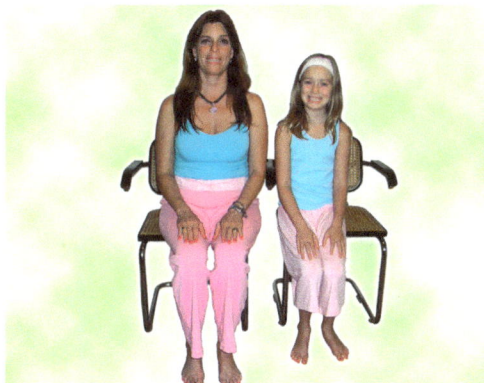

Now, here is the most important step.
Put a big Smile on your face!

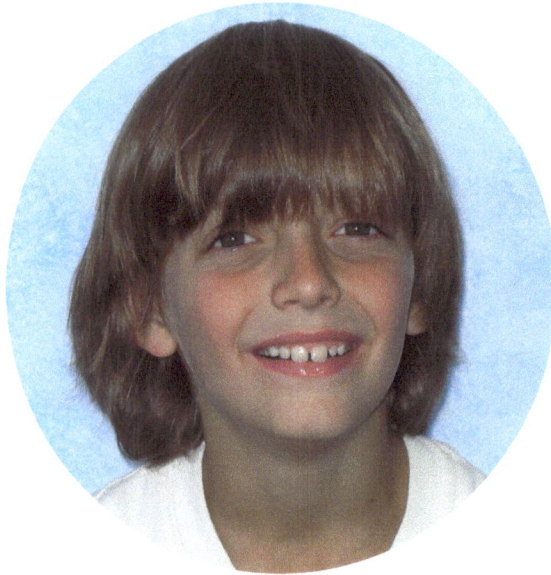

Smile to your Spleen and Pancreas.
Let your Spleen and Pancreas Smile back!

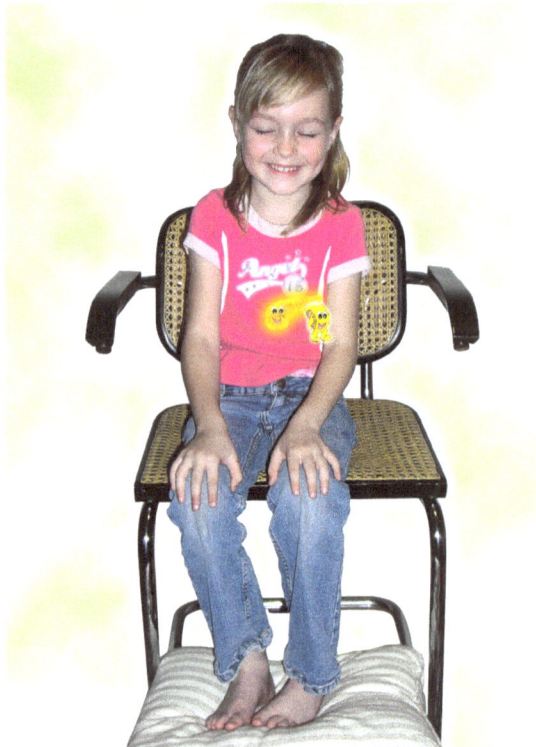

Imagine your Spleen and Pancreas as a beautiful Golden color.

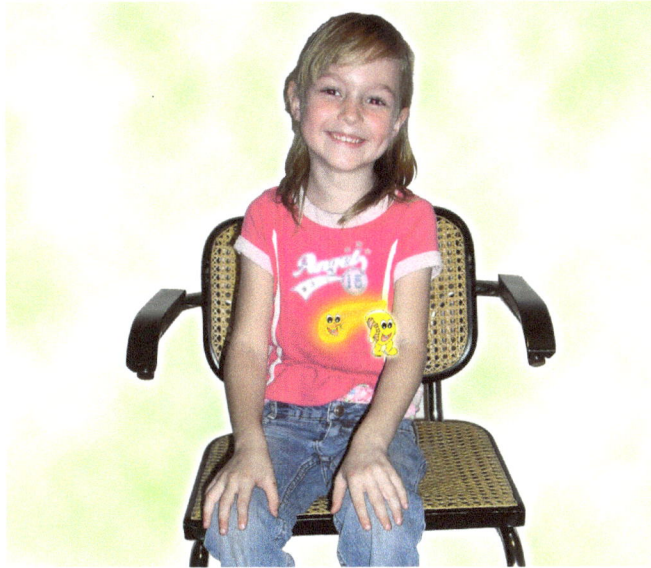

Close your eyes, Smile to your Spleen and Pancreas and breathe in the feelings of Fairness and Openness until you fill your beautiful Golden organs with the Golden color of Fairness and Openness.

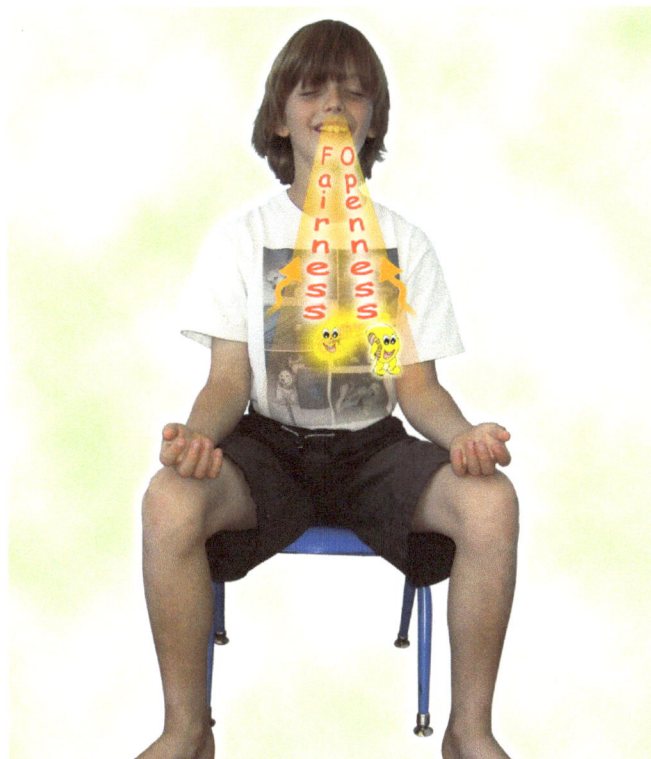

Breathe out the feeling of worry and anxiety (ask your grown up what that anxiety means).

See a dark smoke leave through your mouth and drop down into the earth.

The Earth will take your garbage and use it to grow beautiful things, like flowers or trees.

We call
that transformation.

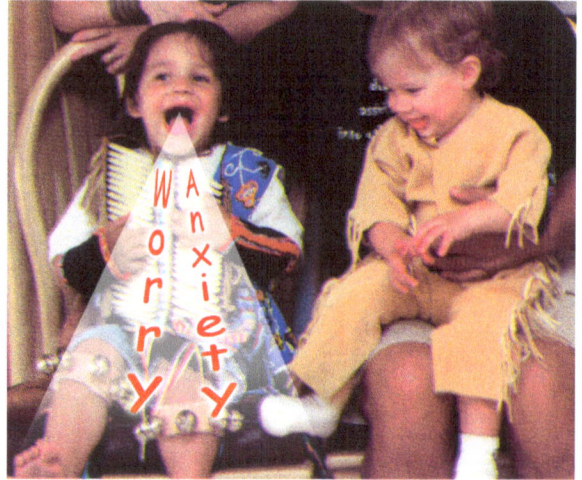

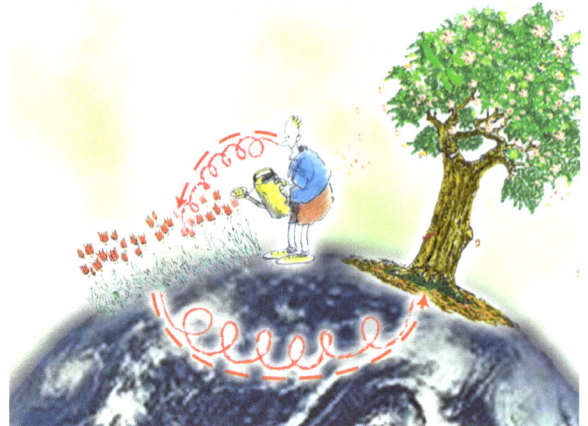

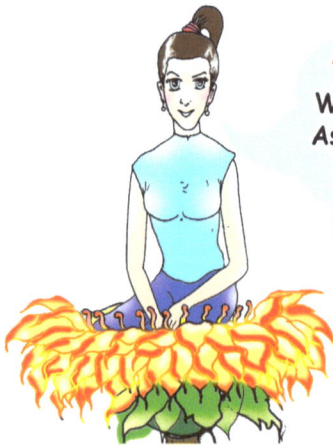

TRANSFORMATION.
Wow! That's a big word.
Ask your grown-up about
that big word.
Bye-bye Anger
Hello flowers.

Smile to your Golden Spleen
and Pancreas.

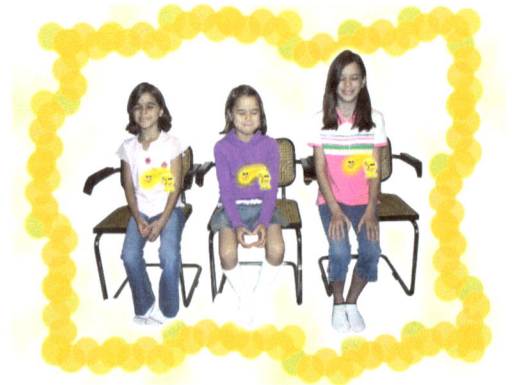

Lets try it again.

This time, we're going to speak to our
Spleen and Pancreas out loud!
The special healing sound of the Spleen
and Pancreas is WHOOO.
Just like the sound an owl makes.

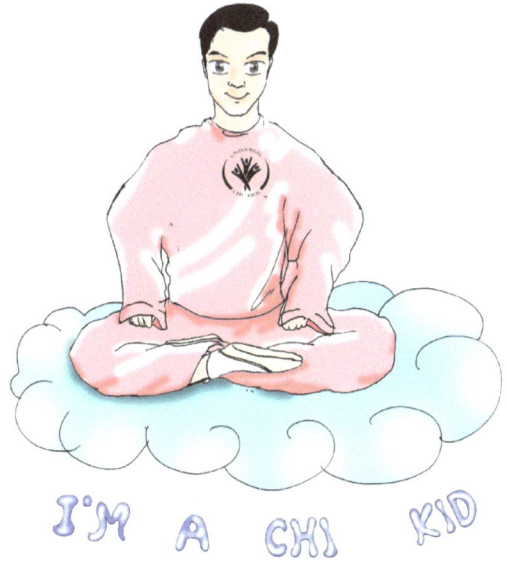

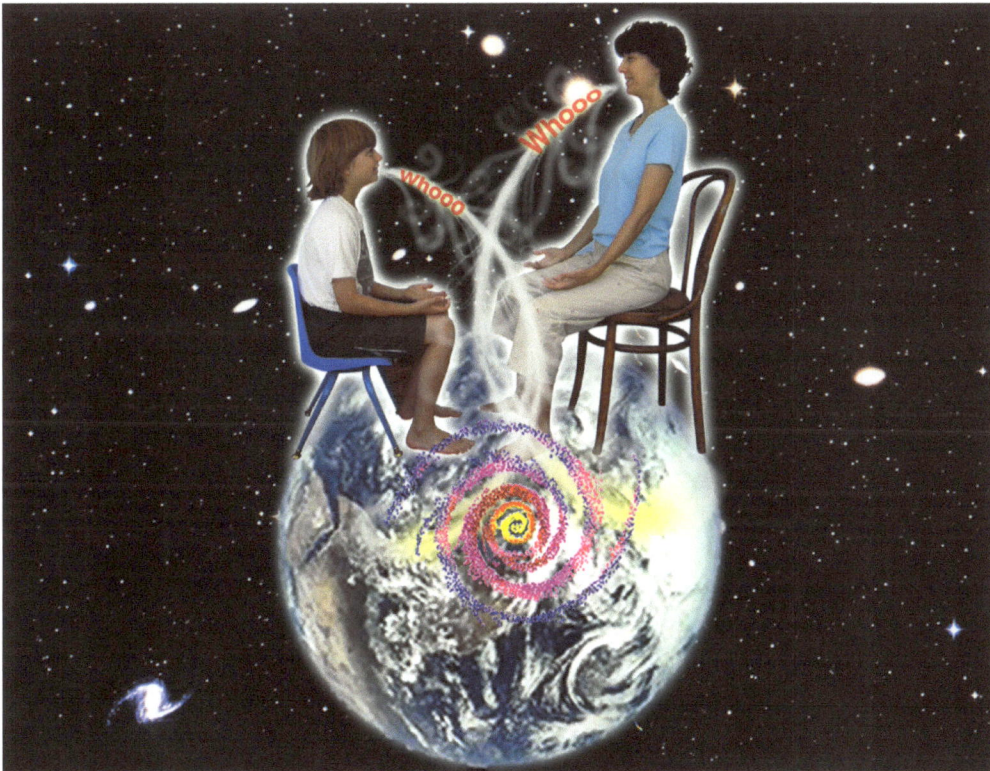

I'M A CHI KID

Can you say WHOOO?

So, now we're going to breathe in Fairness and Openness and breathe out worry and anxiety using the WHOOO sound. Remember to breathe out the dark smoke and let it go into the Earth.

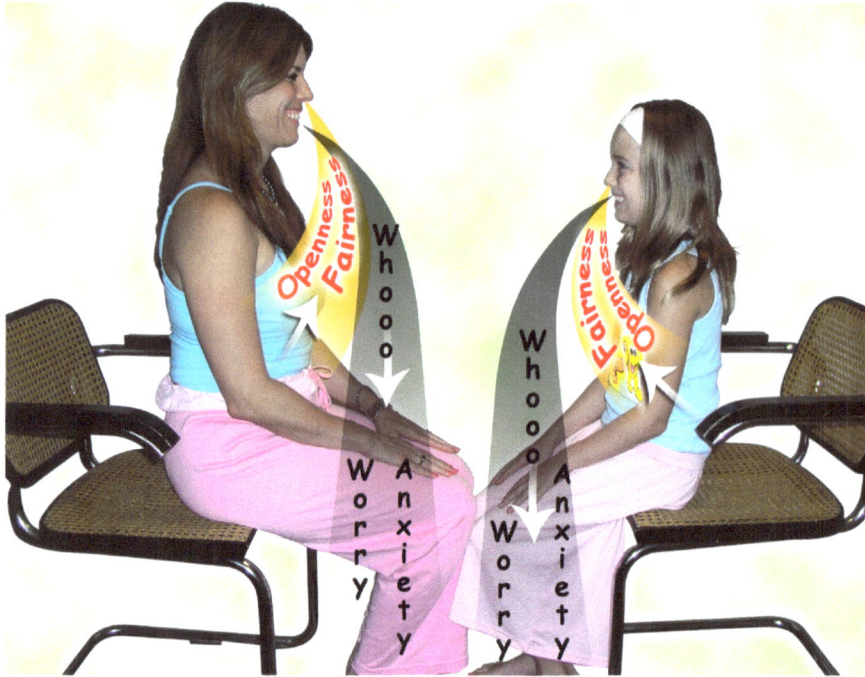

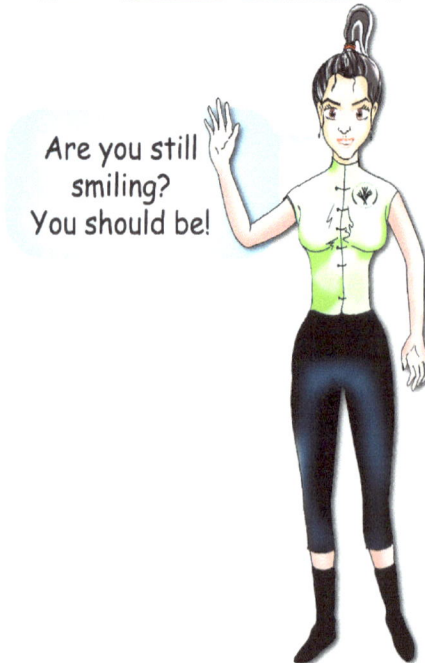

Are you still smiling? You should be!

I'M A CHI KID

Look who's here! It's the Golden Phoenix!

The Golden Phoenix is like a guardian angel for your Spleen and Pancreas.

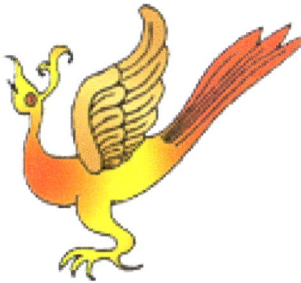

"Hello Mr.Phoenix"

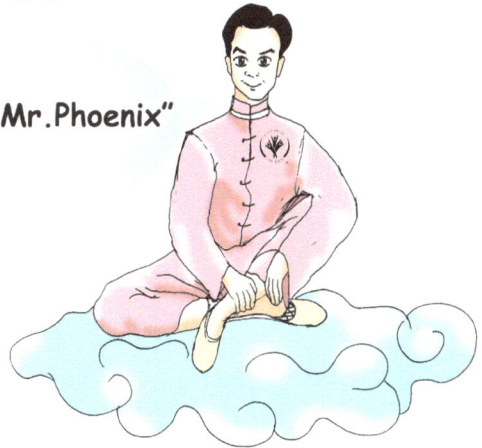

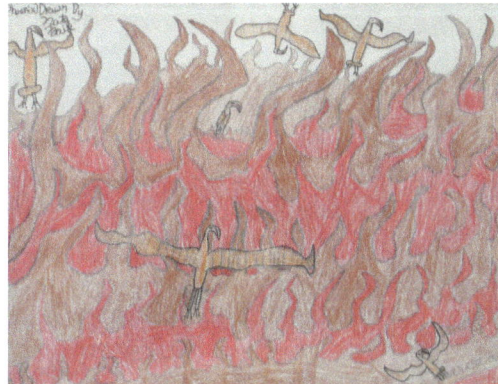

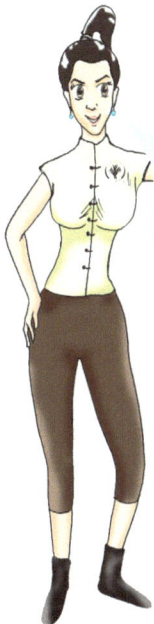

How are you today?

In the Taoist way, we believe there are special animals to protect us from harm. When you Smile to your Golden Spleen and Pancreas, Smile to the Golden Phoenix too!

78

Let's put it all together!
Sit on a chair with your feet on the floor and Smile.
Feel your Spleen and Pancreas and Smile to your Spleen and Pancreas.
See your golden Spleen and Pancreas smile back.
Breathe in Fairness and Openness to your Spleen and Pancreas.
Breath out worry and anxiety using the WHOOOO sound.
Let dark smoke leave your Spleen and Pancreas through your mouth and imagine it sinks into the earth. The Earth can use it to grow something beautiful.
Say "Hello" to the Golden Phoenix that protects your Spleen and Pancreas.
Smile one more time and feel the feelings of Fairness and Openness coming from your Spleen and Pancreas.

Try to do this 3 times in a row!

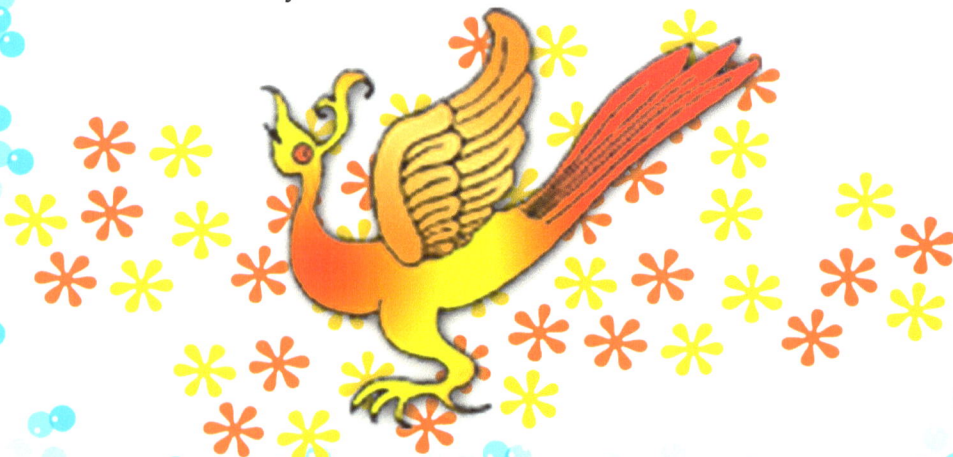

It is always important to take a minute and rest after we smile to our Spleen and Pancreas. Just take one or two minutes and think of how lucky it is that you can share your feelings with the wonderful people in your life and how important it is to be a good and fair friend.

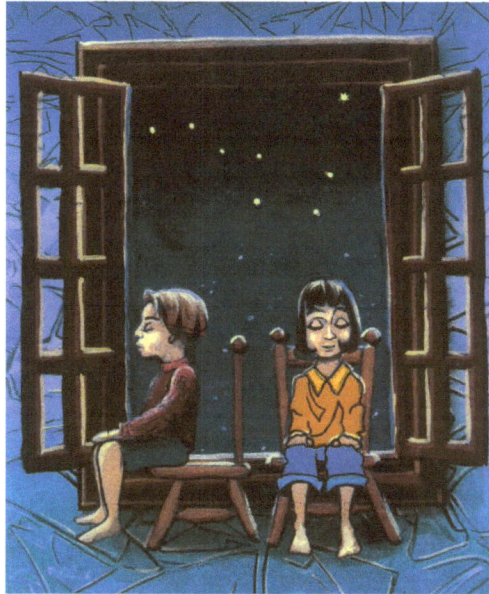

And, remember, always be your best, most honest self.

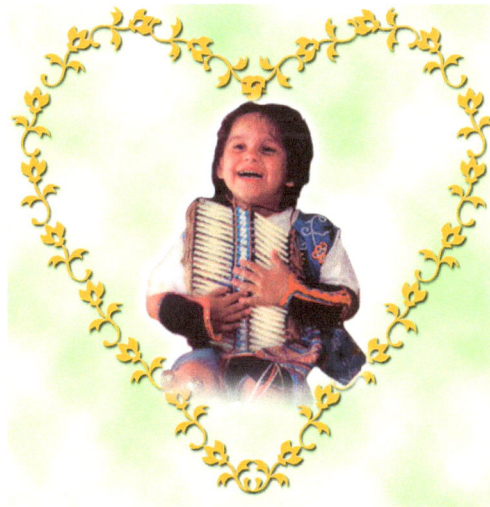

You are a very special person!

Spleen & Pancreas Sound: I can smile to my Spleen & Pancreas

81

www.ingramcontent.com/pod-product-compliance
Lightning Source LLC
Chambersburg PA
CBHW060815270326
41930CB00002B/43